T0211997

'Ending AIDS' in the Age of Biopharmaceuticals

This book considers the change in rhetoric surrounding the treatment of AIDS from one of crisis to that of 'ending AIDS'. Exploring what it means to 'end AIDS' and how responsibility is framed in this new discourse, the author considers the tensions generated between the individual and the state in terms of notions such as risk, responsibility and prevention. Based on analyses and public health promotions in the UK and the US, HIV prevention science and engaging with the work of Foucault, this volume argues that the discourse of 'ending AIDS' implies a tension-filled space in which global principles and values may clash with localized needs, values and concerns; in which evidence-based policies strive for hegemony over local, tacit and communal regimes of knowledge; and in which desires compete with national and international ideas about what is best for the individual in the name of 'ending AIDS' writ large. As such, it will appeal to scholars of sociology and media studies with interests in the sociology of medicine and health, medical communication and health policy.

Tony Sandset is Research Fellow at the Faculty of Medicine at the University of Oslo, Norway, and the author of *Color that Matters: A Comparative Approach to Mixed Race Identity and Nordic Exceptionalism.*

Routledge Studies in the Sociology of Health and Illness

'Ending AIDS' in the Age of Biopharmaceuticals

The Individual, the State and the Politics of Prevention

Tony Sandset

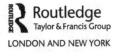
Routledge
Taylor & Francis Group

LONDON AND NEW YORK

First published 2021
by Routledge
2 Park Square, Milton Park, Abingdon, Oxon OX14 4RN

and by Routledge
605 Third Avenue, New York, NY 10017

First issued in paperback 2022

Routledge is an imprint of the Taylor & Francis Group, an informa business

Publisher's Note
The publisher has gone to great lengths to ensure the quality of this reprint but
points out that some imperfections in the original copies may be apparent.

British Library Cataloguing-in-Publication Data
A catalogue record for this book is available from the British Library

Library of Congress Cataloging-in-Publication Data
A catalog record has been requested for this book

ISBN: 978-0-367-52913-0 (pbk)
ISBN: 978-0-367-18583-1 (hbk)
ISBN: 978-0-429-19700-0 (ebk)

DOI: 10.4324/9780429197000

Typeset in Times New Roman
by Deanta Global Publishing Services, Chennai, India

Contents

Acknowledgement

Writing this book has been an immense learning experience, a process of reflection and of introspection and of gazing outwards towards the world. Writing this book would not have been possible without the support, help, and insights provided by friends, colleges and family members. I am indebted to all who have commented upon and given advice on different parts of this book. I am also very grateful to those people who, while not giving direct comments to the book itself, provided invaluable insights and who have shared of their world and of their time.

I am thankful for the people and support at the Faculty of Medicine at the University of Oslo. In particular the KNOWIT research group and Eivind Engebretsen, Kristin Heggen, Gina Henrichsen, Ida Lilleghagen, Clemet Askheim and Carolina Borges Rau Steuernagel. I am also thankful for the insights and advice provided by Kåre Moen and Anne Oleug Olsen at the Institute for Community and Global Health at the University of Oslo.

The process of writing this book has taken me across Europe and the USA, and as such I would like to thank the many people who have provided thoughtful, engaged and critical comments along the way.

I would like to thank Maurice Nagington at the University of Manchester for great insights into PrEP in the context of England. I am thankful for all the thoughtful insights provided by Sara Davis and Ryan Whitacre at the Graduate Institute Geneva. Ian Whitmarsh at UCSF has provided many inspiring comments as well as feedback on various ideas found in this book. At Oxford University, Sara Paparini has provided wonderful help and comments on various ideas that eventually made their way into this book.

I am indebted to Gard Høybjerg for comments and thoughts that he has provided along the way, as well as the insights provided by Victor Shammas.

Alice Salt at Routledge has provided invaluable work and assistance on the production of the book as well as the process leading up to the final product.

I would like to thank Svein and Nadine Hinsch for always coming up with wonderful lessons on how to navigate the past and the present, and who always have provided shelter and recluse when the world storms.

I am indebted to my mother, Judith Sandset. For all that can be expressed in words and for all the things that cannot be expressed by words, I am thankful.

I belong to the belated generation, those who came into adulthood after the AIDS crisis and who perhaps never fully understood the shared impact of the 1980s and 1990s AIDS crisis. As such, I am indebted to those people who came before me, those who continued to fight, to love and to live, in spite of the circumstances they found themselves in. In the spirit of those who have passed, I hope this book might provide some thoughts on the contemporary HIV epidemic so that the future might be conceptualized differently.

Finally, this book then, is dedicated more than anything else to those who have passed in the HIV epidemic, and those who keep living with HIV, those who keep loving, those who keep being vocal about the issues that still haunt the global HIV efforts and those who insist that the future might hold different ways of living with and near HIV. I hope my small contribution to such a conceptualization of the future will bear at least some fruits when this book is read.

Glossary

PrEP	Pre Exposure Prophylaxis
UNAIDS	Joint United Nations Programme on HIV/AIDS
PEPFAR	President's Emergency Plan for AIDS Relief.
NHS	National Health Services
HIV	Human Immunodeficiency Virus
AIDS	Acquired Immune Deficiency Syndrome
ARV	Antiretroviral drugs
ART	Antiretroviral Therapy
TasP	Treatment as Prevention

Part I

Setting the stage for the end of AIDS

1   Introduction

> Eradicate. to destroy completely; put an end to. From Latin, eradicate – torn up by the root.
>
> – Oxford Online Dictionary

This book starts with the question of what it means to 'end AIDS', to 'eradicate it once and for all'? It starts from the realization that there seems to have been a profound shift in how the HIV epidemic is framed. Former UNAIDS Executive Director Michel Sidibe stated in 2014 'Ending AIDS is an opportunity for this generation. We should not miss this opportunity' (UNAIDS, 2014a). Fast forward to 2018, when New York City Mayor, Bill de Blasio, stated, 'Reaching our goal to end the AIDS epidemic by 2020 in New York City is a good start, but we won't rest until we eradicate the epidemic once and for all' (De Blasio, 2018). This new framing of the end of AIDS seems almost omnipresent; the notion that 'we' can end AIDS sooner rather than later can be found in global health strategies made by UNAIDS and in the strategies and reports made by the President's Emergency Plan for AIDS Relief (PEPFAR), the largest donor of HIV funding to low- and middle-income countries (LMIC). It can be found within the media promotions of private pharmaceutical companies such as Gilead Sciences in their video promotion *Gilead HIV: HIV Ends with Us*.[1] It has found its way to national HIV strategies, such as the current White House strategy aptly named *Ending the HIV Epidemic: A Plan for America* (HIV.gov, 2019). Finally, it has come to be a slogan for a multitude of local-, state- and city-based HIV campaigns in the US and Europe. A few examples would be the multimedia campaign *HIV Stops with Me* based in the US,[2] the *It Starts with Me* campaign based in England[3] and the *Be Sure, Play Sure, Stay Sure* campaign based in New York City (NYCDOH, 2020).

However, what does ending AIDS entail? Who will be ending it and how? Where will the end come about and when will AIDS be ended? If ending something signifies the final part of a period of time, an activity or a story, then what does this signify in terms of the end of AIDS? Finally, since the HIV epidemic is, to a large degree, an epidemic driven by social inequality and health inequity, does the end of AIDS also signify the end of inequality?

These questions open up too many avenues for thought and too many optics for a critical engagement with the end of AIDS. However, I want to engage with how the end of AIDS can be made problematic; that is, the very notion of the end of AIDS should be approached not as a solution to a problem, but rather as a problem unto itself. The end of AIDS, I postulate, is an assemblage of productive meaning-making, of continual action and the generating of new signifying practices of what it means to end AIDS. Paula Treichler, writing in 1999, stated 'the AIDS epidemic has produced a parallel epidemic of meanings, definitions and attributions. This semantic epidemic, which I have come to call an *epidemic of signification*, has not diminished in the 1990s' (Treichler, 1999:1). In many ways, the discourse of ending AIDS is also an epidemic of signification; that is, the end of AIDS narrative keeps producing meanings, definitions and attributions, all of which are concerned in one way or another with the problem of how to end AIDS.

To be more specific for the reader, this book focuses on *how the notion of ending AIDS* has emerged within the last ten years. Secondly, and building from the history that has enabled the slogan 'ending AIDS' to emerge, I want to focus on two themes that have emerged within the current end of AIDS discourse. The first is a reemerging of the importance of geography and space as an important avenue for HIV surveillance, intervention and preventive efforts. The second is the continual focus on key populations and, in particular, on men who have sex with men (MSM) and transgender women.

While specific places and key populations have long been focal points within the HIV epidemic, I want to highlight how the 'end of AIDS' discourse has increasingly come to rely on biomedical and technological interventions as tools for reaching the end of AIDS. This book is about how certain spaces and networks have come to be made or configured through surveillance technology as spaces of risk and transmission, of interventions and control. Secondly, the book also follows up on how Kane Race, in his book *The Gay Science* (Race, 2017:20), investigated how MSM have been 'made into responsible subjects of HIV prevention and harm reduction at different historical moments and through different assemblages'. I want to follow up on this here and look at how the very notion of the end of AIDS also highlights space, place and key populations concerning the various assemblages of biomedical technologies of treatment and prevention.

I should, here at the outset, clarify the title of the book as well as the relationship between HIV and AIDS. The book's title is linked to the slogan 'ending AIDS' which has emerged within the last ten years or so. It has found its linguistic expression through monikers such as 'ending AIDS', or 'ending the epidemic' and 'getting to zero'. However, it is important to note that the slogan 'ending AIDS' is a somewhat different goal than ending HIV. I will be using 'ending AIDS' as a shorthand for ending the epidemic in this book, as it more clearly will highlight the goal of many of the strategies and technologies analyzed in this book. However, as is well known, AIDS is not HIV. HIV is the virus, while AIDS is a medical condition that is the result of an untreated HIV infection once several medical criteria are fulfilled. Ending AIDS as such is more a metonym for the broader notion that both HIV and AIDS will be ended through various interventions. Yet, the linguistic ecology that is circulating is diverse. Ending AIDS is but one of many monikers. Some of them include monikers such as 'getting to zero' which alludes to zero new HIV infections as well as zero new deaths due to AIDS. Another slogan used by PEPFAR is 'an HIV-free generation' which highlights the work done toward a future where no new HIV infections will be seen. Finally, there is the general phrase of 'ending the epidemic' which can be read as both alluding to ending the HIV epidemic and, in connection to this, AIDS. For the sake of clarity and consistency, I have chosen to focus on the phrase of 'ending AIDS' as a way of talking about the general effort to reduce, limit, control or even eradicate HIV.

In a sense, this book is about how what Kane Race has called 'HIV science' (Race, 2017:2) engages with the problematization of how to end AIDS. It is a book about how HIV science problematizes space and populations and how recent biomedical and technological solutions are being researched, framed and mediated as part of the cultural chronicling of the end of AIDS. Kane Race stated that his work in *The Gay Science* was 'about the *risks* and *pleasures* of HIV science – its involvement in the production of situations it cannot anticipate, its capacity to reorganize social and material worlds' (Race, 2017:2). In doing this, Race investigated the 'encounter between HIV social science and the sexual practices of gay and other men who have sex with men in the urban centers of Australia, concerning similar developments in Europe, USA and Canada' (Race, 2017:2). My contribution is similar, yet different. This book is about how HIV science is involved with the production of the narrative of ending AIDS through its focus on biomedical and technological innovations meant to contribute to the end of AIDS. How HIV science aimed at ending, eradicating or controlling the HIV epidemic reorganizes spatial, social and material worlds as well as subjectivities.

I do this through an analysis that will be focusing, like Race, on how HIV science encounters spaces and communities of men who have sex with men and other key populations in the USA and Europe, with some references to other global sites. Again, like Race, my claim is that the end of AIDS narrative as we see it unfold in the spaces I just mentioned is highly predicated upon an intense focus on the behavior of MSM as well as certain hotspots or spaces that are of particular focus in ending AIDS. However, I do not mean to say that the problematization of the end of AIDS unfolds only through pervasive social control and surveillance, a warning that Kane Race also makes (Race, 2017:3). I want to offer a cultural chronicling of how MSM communities and other key populations have subverted, reacted to and resisted the many biomedical and technological interventions meant to reform communities in the name of ending AIDS. If Paula Treichler offered a cultural chronicle of the beginning of the HIV/AIDS epidemic, and if Nora Kenworthy and Matthew Thomann opened up a critical inquiry into what the end of AIDS might signify, then my contribution is perhaps a cultural chronicle of how the end of AIDS discourse has emerged as a signifying epidemic.

The drive to end AIDS rests on several premises, many of them embedded in a firm belief in biomedical and technological interventions, such as increased HIV testing rates, the scale-up and rollout of antiretroviral treatment (ARV) drugs for people living with HIV (PLHIV), increased reliance on pre-exposure prophylaxis (PrEP) for people who are at high risk of contracting HIV, as well as enhanced HIV surveillance methods, such as viral load maps and HIV transmission mapping through so-called 'phylogenetic testing'. On top of this, mathematical modeling of transmission rates, treatment coverage and testing uptakes have come to occupy increasingly central positions within epidemiological modeling, alleging to show the way toward the end of AIDS.

All of these technologies are in some way framed as being answers to the problem of HIV and the road to ending AIDS. Yet the argument in this book is that while these are important pieces on the road to controlling the HIV epidemic, these interventions themselves can be seen not as solutions but rather as answers to a particular way of envisioning the HIV epidemic as a specific form of problem. In doing so, this invites us to critically interrogate the taken-for-granted notion that these technologies and biomedical solutions are answers to the problem of HIV.

Rather than starting from the idea that the end of AIDS is the *solution to the problem of the HIV epidemic*, I want to invert this and think about the end of AIDS as a *problematic* – a problem rather than a solution. In doing so, I want to provide what Paula Treichler has called 'a cultural chronicle' of the HIV epidemic (Treichler, 1999). Treichler, writing in 1999 and chronicling the beginning of the HIV epidemic, provides us with an invaluable premise when she states that the HIV epidemic is just as much an 'epidemic of signification' or an epidemic of meaning as it is an infectious disease epidemic. Following Treichler, I want to provide a cultural chronicle, not of the beginning of the HIV epidemic, but its end – the discourse and politics of an era that envisions that the end of AIDS is within reach.

This book starts from a very particular moment in the history of the HIV/AIDS epidemic and then uses this moment as its starting point for an investigation into the very phrase of 'ending AIDS'. The historical moment I refer to is the launch of the UNAIDS Fast Track strategy in 2014 (UNAIDS, 2014a). From this historic event, I go mostly forward, but I also trace some of the conditions of the emergence of this strategy as a necessary precondition to understanding the current narrative of the end of AIDS.

As part of this, I also want to highlight the 2016 UNAIDS adoption of the *Political Declaration on HIV and AIDS: On the Fast Track to Accelerate the Fight against HIV and to Ending the AIDS Epidemic by 2030* (UNAIDS, 2014b). In the Declaration, the heads of states pledged to 'reaffirm our commitment to end the AIDS epidemic by 2030 as our legacy to present and future generations, to accelerate and scale up the fight against HIV and end AIDS to reach this target' (UNAIDS, 2016). Furthermore, the Declaration stated that 'HIV and AIDS continue to constitute a global emergency, pose one of the most formidable challenges to the development, progress, and stability of our respective societies and the world at large; and require an exceptional and comprehensive global response' (UNAIDS, 2016). The Declaration pledged that adopting the UNAIDS' '90-90-90 targets' and reaching them by 2020 would ensure that 'no one would be left behind' on the road to end AIDS by 2030 (UNAIDS, 2016). The Declaration builds heavily on this 90-90-90 fast track strategy developed by UNAIDS and stipulates that '90% of people living with HIV know their HIV status; 90% of people who know their status receive treatment; 90% of people on HIV treatment have a suppressed viral load' (UNAIDS, 2014a).

Seeing that recent research has firmly established that people with a suppressed viral load live close to normal life expectancy if started on treatment early (Harris, Rabkin, & El-Sadr, 2018; Trickey et al., 2017) and are unable to transmit HIV onward (Anthony & Fauci, 2019; Eisinger, Dieffenbach, & Fauci, 2019), the goal of viral suppression has become both the end goal of clinical care for people living with HIV (PLHIV) and an important public health indicator.

In the aftermath of the adoption of the declaration to accelerate the efforts to end AIDS by the UN, the 90-90-90 targets have become part of many nations' public health response toward ending AIDS. Many nations now use these indicators as a way of reporting the progress on ending AIDS and thus fulfilling the global promise made in the UN's Sustainable Development Goals (SDGs) on 'ending AIDS' and ensuring an 'HIV-free generation'. UNAIDS states that 'When this three-part target is achieved, at least 73% of all people living with HIV worldwide will be virally suppressed – a two- to three-fold increase over current rough estimates of viral suppression' (UNAIDS, 2014a:3). As such, there has been an immense drive to roll out various HIV treatment and prevention efforts all in the name of ending AIDS through the achievement of globally reaching the 90-90-90 targets. Several international stakeholders have started to subscribe to the idea that not only is the end of AIDS a possibility, but it is also an imminent event (Sidibé, Loures, & Samb, 2016; UNAIDS, 2014a). Conversely, it should be mentioned that other actors within the global HIV effort use variations of these goals. PEPFAR uses a variant based on what they have modeled to be 'epidemic control' (PEPFAR, 2017). The UN's SDGs use a slightly different indicator, which is a number of new HIV infections per 100,000 (UN Agenda 2030, 2015). In all cases, the end goal or success criteria is inevitably linked to the reduction in new cases, which is often linked to a communal reduction of viral load measures.

However, recent reports have shown that even with the dramatic shift in the historical trajectory of HIV, there are still vast gaps in access to treatment and care as well as large geographical and demographic differences in terms of access to testing, treatment and retention within the treatment cascade (UNAIDS 2018a, 2018b). UNAIDS has also warned about complacency concerning the HIV epidemic, cautioning that inability to scale up efforts will delay or reverse progress, and may exacerbate the epidemic, particularly in terms of key population groups, such as transgender women, women of color, people who inject drugs, sex workers and men who have sex with men (UNAIDS, 2018a). The HIV epidemic is still a major global health concern, and its impact is still felt across the globe, oftentimes in highly disproportionate ways. UNAIDS numbers show us that there still are between 640,000 and 1.3 million who die of AIDS-related causes each year globally and between 1.4 million and 2.4 million new HIV infections each year.[4]

Donor funding has plateaued or diminished in spite of calls for increased funding from donor countries in an attempt to scale up the UNAIDS fast track strategy (Kenworthy, Thomann, & Parker, 2018a, 2018b; UNAIDS, 2018a). So what then does it mean to end AIDS within the current climate of both broad optimism that the end of AIDS is within reach and, on the other hand, the all too present acknowledgment that there still are, as UNAIDS states, 'miles to go' (UNAIDS, 2018a) until the end of AIDS is ensured?

Within the strange tension between the hope that the HIV epidemic can be controlled and potentially ended, and, on the other hand, a sense of a 'prevention crisis' as well as a 'funding crisis' (UNAIDS, 2018a), an increased focus has been on scaling up and utilizing several new biomedical and technological innovations. I argue that biomedical interventions, as they are rolled out and represented, can be seen as answers to a particular framing of the problem of HIV; thus the answer they provide must inevitably be shaped by how the problem of HIV has been framed in the first place. This becomes particularly poignant concerning power and politics in global health. Power and politics in this new era of the 90-90-90 targets have shifted, this book postulates, toward a mixture of 'audit culture' (Shore & Wright, 2015), neo-liberalization of both public health and global health aid, and a push toward a governmentality which relies upon an increased use of metrics and indicators that allows for a 'governance of self-governance' (Miller & Rose, 2008, 2017).

To this end, the current historical moment in the HIV epidemic has become dominated by an immense focus, both scholarly and politically, on the biomedical aspects of the end of AIDS as well as the economic aspects of what it will take to end AIDS. As Susan Kippax and Niamh Stephenson argues, since around 1996–1997, there has been an immense 'biomedical turn' within the global HIV effort (Kippax & Stephenson, 2016). This biomedical turn has become more and more dominant with the introduction of the 90-90-90 targets and novel drug candidates. While the biomedical turn has been important in reducing mortality, extending life expectancies for people living with HIV as well as offering prophylactic protection to people at risk of HIV infections, Kippax and Stephenson argue differently. They note that until the day that biomedicine develops an effective vaccine and a cure for the millions of people living with HIV, we must not forget the social and cultural aspects of the HIV epidemic (Kippax & Stephenson, 2016:1). The same point has been noted by several scholars such as anthropologist Didier Fassin (Fassin, 2007), anthropologist and medical doctor Vinh-Kim Nguyen (Nguyen, 2010; Nguyen, O'Malley, & Pirkle, 2011) and anthropologist and medical doctor Paul Farmer (Farmer, 2006). In following the work of these eminent scholars, this book on the end of AIDS and what it entails seeks not so much to engage with the effectiveness of the 90-90-90 targets nor the political economy of cost-effectiveness. Rather I want to inquire how theory can be used in analyzing the end of AIDS as an epidemic of signification.

How to have theory at the end of AIDS?

As should be clear by now, this book seeks to look at how the end of AIDS narrative has fostered a new 'epidemic of signification' (Kenworthy et al., 2018a,

2018b; Treichler, 1999). As Paula Treichler noted in her seminal work *How to have theory in an epidemic. Cultural chronicles of AIDS* (Treichler, 1999), the AIDS epidemic is cultural and linguistic as well as biological and biomedical (Treichler, 1999:1). To understand the HIV epidemic's history, address its future and learn from its lessons, we must take Treichler's assertion seriously. Treichler sought to understand the AIDS epidemic through a careful examination of language and culture that she asserted, would enable us to think carefully about ideas amid a crisis, and that this critical thinking through and with the cultural and linguistic signifying practices during the AIDS epidemic would allow us to consider both theoretical problems, develop policy and articulate long-term social needs (Treichler, 1999:1). If Treichler sought to encouraged us to think critically on the role of culture and language during a time of AIDS crisis, then my contribution is to ask us to think critically on the role and function of the language of biomedicine and technology in an era that professes to be close to ending AIDS and in a post-crisis world. My argument is that the new focus on a biomedical and technologically driven end of AIDS can be analyzed as also creating a 'parallel epidemic of meanings, definitions and attributions' (Treichler, 1999:1). The need for an analysis of the current epidemic of signification in an era that professes to soon end AIDS seems more relevant than ever. Treichler emphasized that in AIDS, meanings are overwhelming in their sheer volume and often explicitly linked to extreme political agendas (Treichler, 1999:39). This led Treichler to state that what we need is

> an epidemiology of signification – a comprehensive mapping and analysis of these multiple meanings – to form the basis for an official definition that will, in turn, constitute the policies, regulations, rules and practices that will govern our behavior for some time to come.
>
> (Treichler, 1999:39)

Kenworthy et al., writing in 2018, states that

> now more than ever, Treichler's arguments ring true as we reflect critically on the discursive construction of the 'end of AIDS' narrative in recent years – and on how this narrative has shaped policies and practices that constitute the response to HIV mid-way through the fourth decade of the epidemic.
>
> (Kenworthy et al., 2018b:962)

This book follows in the footsteps of Treichler while also paying attention to the work of, for instance, Kenworthy et al. in offering an analysis of how the end of AIDS narrative has ushered in a new, or perhaps modified, epidemic of signification as Paula Treichler might have said.

In this new epidemic of signification, we can ask, as Kenworthy et al. do,

> What does the end of AIDS signify and for whom? Who stands to benefit from a triumphalism that few believe, but many endorse? And most importantly,

what kind of AIDS response does this discourse promote and what forms of knowledge is it rooted in?

(Kenworthy et al., 2018b:962)

Phrased differently, we might ask 'Where, how and for whom AIDS might be ending?' (Benton, Sangaramoorthy, & Kalofonos, 2017:474), and conversely, 'Where, how and for whom the end of the epidemic is a far more distant hope?' (Kenworthy et al., 2018a:958). Connecting this more concretely to this book's main concerns, we might ask how the end of AIDS discourse, its knowledge practices and its cultural and linguistic signifying practices also predicates a certain way of problematizing the end of AIDS. If cultural and linguistic signifying practices are key in order to understand what kind of end to AIDS we are witnessing, to who this end might come, where it will come and how it will come, then this book argues that a large part of this is predicated upon a specific form of making HIV and AIDS problematic.

To speak of the end of AIDS, as an epidemic of signification might seem to move the focus from the practice of ending AIDS to the theory of ending AIDS, which might strike some as engaging in intellectual sophistry and ignoring the often deadly and painful realities of the HIV epidemic. However, an analysis of the end of AIDS as a specific form of problematization is far from just a form of theoretical sophistry.

The late Stuart Hall formulated it well when he first raised the question of how we could bridge the gap between a form of cultural studies analysis of the AIDS epidemic and the practical reality of the very same epidemic wherein people were dying. Hall asked,

> Against the urgency of people dying in the streets, what in God's name is the point of cultural studies? What is the point of the study of representation if there is no response to the question of what you say to someone who wants to know if they should take a drug and if that means they'll die two days later or a few months later?

(Hall, 1996:271)

The question is pertinent and still important. For Hall, this question must have weighed heavily upon him as he went on to say that

> I think anybody who is into cultural studies seriously as an intellectual practice must feel, on their pulse, its ephemerality, its insubstantiality, how little it registers, how little we've been able to change anything or get anybody to do anything.

(Hall, 1996:271)

While this seems to border on a sort of surrender or even exhaustion, Hall nevertheless reaffirms the use, the dignity and the critical value of an analysis of AIDS through cultural studies when he later states

How could we say that the question of AIDS is not also a question of who gets represented and who does not? AIDS is the site at which the advance of sexual politics is being rolled back [...] Unless we operate within this tension [between the biomedical and the social, between the practical and the theoretical], we don't know what cultural studies can do, can't, never can do; but also, what it has to do, what it alone has the privileged capacity to do.

(Hall, 1996:272)

Paula Treichler followed the words of Hall by stating that an analysis of the cultural chronicles of the AIDS epidemic could help us understand the complex relationship between language and reality, between meanings and definitions – and how those relations help us understand AIDS and develop interventions that are more culturally informed and socially responsible (Treichler, 1999:4). I would like to add to Hall and Treichler that to write a book about the end of AIDS, as a form of cultural analysis of the present moment of the HIV epidemic, offers a way of looking at how the end of AIDS discourse has ushered in new ways of thinking problematically around HIV and that these new signifying practices indeed play on a new set of power regimes which facilitate and constrain our ability to think about the end of AIDS.

The problem of HIV and the problematization of the end of AIDS

I have already stated that this book seeks to engage with a critical analysis of what the end of AIDS means; that is, for whom the end of AIDS is a reality, where will it end, the way will it end and what this end will signify in the political and semiotic economy of lived lives. The starting point for this critical engagement is simply the emergence of a very palpable discourse across the globe that we can end AIDS by 2030 as, for instance, the UN sustainable development goals (SDGs) stipulates. However, rather than starting from the assumption that the end of AIDS discourse is the answer to the problem of HIV/AIDS, I want to approach the very notion of an end to AIDS from the perspective of *problematization* as it figures in the work of Michel Foucault (1984b, 2001), that of Carol Bacchi (Bacchi, 2012, 2015; Bacchi & Goodwin, 2016) and, to a certain degree, of Gilles Deleuze (1994).

So, what does it mean to think problematically about the end of AIDS? What specific vantage points does this give us in terms of thinking about the signifying practices of the current drive to end AIDS? To answer this question, I want to give an account of the theoretical and methodological influences that structures my notion of thinking problematically about the end of AIDS. So, how to think problematically about the end of AIDS? Conversely, what is it that the end of AIDS is an answer to? What is the problem of HIV/AIDS? On the surface of it, the end of AIDS and its many biomedical and technological interventions seems to be an answer to a global epidemic that has been ongoing since at least 1981 and has claimed the lives of 32 million people since its start.[5] Currently,

37.9 million people are living with HIV at the end of 2018 (UNAIDS, 2019), and between 570,000 and 1.1 million people died of AIDS-related diseases in 2018. In light of these numbers and the gravity of the epidemic both historically and currently, the end of AIDS seems to provide us with an answer to limit and halt onwards HIV transmissions, to provide ARVs to all who need it and to offer HIV testing to as many as possible as well as providing care and treatment for people living with HIV.

Yet, in light of this, what will a problematization of the end of AIDS provide us? For one, we can start by asking what does it mean to think problematically around HIV/AIDS? What were the preconditions that allowed for this very concept to emerge in the specific form that it did and through what modalities has it taken form? Foucault states that the study of various practices should start from a study of 'problematization', that is asking, 'how and why certain things (behavior, phenomena, processes) became a problem' (Michel Foucault, 2001:171). In investigating various problems, Foucault states that there is a certain double movement to the study of problematization; that is, one tries in the same analytical frame to 'see how the different solutions to a problem have been constructed; but also, how these solutions result from a specific form of problematization' (Michel Foucault, 1984a:389). Such a starting point might be to think about the discourse of ending AIDS not as a solution, but, indeed, as a answer to a problem – to the problem of HIV/AIDS. However, we should be careful not to think that ending AIDS is a banal answer to the *problem of AIDS*, rather, linking the concept of problematization to the discourse of AIDS means not just looking at it as a reply to a question, that is, 'what to do about AIDS?'

As Michael Warner warns us, the usage of the term 'problematization' is not just to view something as a historically contingent problem: the

> term, awkward enough under the best of circumstances, has become rather confused by its use among post-Foucauldian academics, for whom it often means nothing more than taking something to be problematic. To problematize, in this usage, means to complicate.
>
> (Warner, 2002:125–158)

Rather, following Warner again, we can state that the issue of problematization has a much richer meaning which Warner traces back to Foucault's work on the *History of Sexuality Volume 2* and *Volume 3* (Michel Foucault, 2012a, 2012b). As Warner states,

> There, he (Foucault) treats a problematic not just as an intellectual tangle, but also as the practical horizon of intelligibility within which problems come to matter for people. It stands for both the conditions that make thinking possible and for the way thinking, under certain circumstances, can reflect on its conditions. Problematization is more than arguing; it is a practical context for thinking. As such, it lies largely beyond conscious strategy.
>
> (Warner, 2002:154–155)

As such, problematization is deeply connected to people's everyday lives; it is directly connected to the practical manners in which people conduct their own lives and how they relate to the problems in their lives, the obstacles and practical realities of their lives.

Problematization as Foucault used it, shuttles back and forth between two poles: the first is problematization as 'an object of analysis. For example, the process by which modes of living or modes of self-care become problems is what is meant by problematization'.[6] In this form, problematization is seen through the well-known formulation made by Foucault that problematization is the name given to the development of a genealogy of problems. Foucault notes that we should pay attention to 'Why a problem and why such a kind of problem, why a certain way of problematizing appears at a given point in time' (M. Foucault, Lotringer, & Hochroth, 2007:141). The history of the HIV/AIDS epidemic is rife with problems to which we have responded, but as I will argue later on and build on the work of Kane Race (Race, 2017), the problematization of HIV/AIDS is not just an answer to how to end AIDS or ensure an HIV-free generation. Rather, I will argue that the problem of HIV/AIDS as the practical context for thinking is also about the problem of sex and intimacy. It is about the ordering of knowledge about human intimacy, how to know it, to account for it and to control it. It's about answering the perceived problem of sex and its relationship to human behavior, conduct and practice.

Going back to the term problematization and its usage as an optic for analysis, we should note that the above-mentioned way of looking at problematization is highly popular in governmentality studies as well as actor-network studies. Here problematization is taken to be a process of framing in which problems are defined in ways that enroll various partners and shape subsequent pathways of action, decision, inquiry and intervention (Barnett, 2019). Thus, problematization seeks to answer why a certain problem arose at a particular moment in time, what ways in which this particular problem has been suggested solved, and, perhaps above all, how human conduct has been shaped by this problem – what ethical, practical and material responses have been given to this problem through its many modes of forming human conduct. Already here we can see that the problematization of HIV/AIDS can be fit quite firmly within such an analytical frame as this. Furthermore, the problematization of ending AIDS is not just an answer to a problem but becomes itself an object of problematization, a key point in this book going forward.

As stated, problematization shuttles between two poles as an analytical model of looking at an object. We have already discerned the first one above and, as such, the second one should also be accounted for. In this second mode, the presumption is that problematization is more of a procedure to be followed by researchers (Barnett, 2019). The attraction of this interpretation is that it aligns quite easily with the idea that the task of analysis is primarily to call into question taken-for-granted assumptions and identities and settlements. As Raymond Geuss formulates it, problematization in this sense aligns well with an understanding of critique as 'putting into question, or as a way of problematizing something'

(Geuss, 2002:211). In this view, problematization as an analytical tool is geared toward unpacking the taken-for-granted assumptions about how the world ordinarily hangs together. Geuss states: 'The principal targets of this problematizing approach are the self-evident assumptions of a given form of life and the (supposedly) natural or inevitable and unchangeable character of given identities' (Geuss, 2002:221). The ending of AIDS seems self-evident. It is a trope that various actors can align themselves around and rally support for, yet its modes of *ending* AIDS seems to have not yet been critically examined as historically contingent modes of thinking the *end* with. That is one of the arguments that will be made in this book: neoliberal ideas, such as personal responsibility for one's health, have become increasingly dominant, and market choice of HIV preventive technologies have been pushed as one means of ending AIDS. Finally, that the end of AIDS seems to rest on a firm biomedicalization of HIV wherein there might be a danger of pushing to the side and out of view larger structural and social issues that are drivers of the epidemic.

The two modes in which we can invoke the term problematization as both a noun and a verb can thus be seen as offering a useful duality in looking at the end of AIDS as a historical narrative as much as it is an ongoing slogan to which actors can rally around. The two senses of problematization easily support a model in which the critical task is presumed to be one of exposing the contingencies of supposedly naturalized formations (Barnett, 2019). In this usage, problematization is used to refer, firstly, to the idea that certain problems that appear to be naturally given or objective are the effects of historical processes, social practices and political strategies. Problematization, in this first sense, is an object of analysis. Secondly, is the assumption that the task of critical analysis is to expose the contingency of apparently stable and taken-for-granted definitions of problems. Problematization, in this second sense, is a prerogative of the critic as the active subject of revelatory truth. In this sense, thinking problematically about the end of AIDS, requires us to think of contingency as a relational quality rather than a fact to be demonstrated, so that the task of analysis becomes one of clarifying the conditions and situations to which problems are a response (Koopman, 2011:1–12). In responding to this claim from Koopman, we can tentatively state that one of the key issues in this book will be to clarify the conditions from which the very term 'ending AIDS' arose, what were and are the contingencies from whence the end of AIDS could be discerned and what have been the problematic situations that the end of AIDS as a public health discourse has tried to respond to?

In linking this to Foucault's terms, we can look at a quote from Foucault when he states that how the concept of problematization works is by the work it does to

> rediscover at the root of these diverse solutions the general form of problematization that has made them possible – even in their very opposition; or what has made possible the transformations of the difficulties and obstacles of a practice into a general problem for which one proposes diverse practical solutions. It is problematization that responds to these difficulties, but by doing something quite other than expressing them or manifesting them: in

connection with them, it develops the conditions in which possible response will be given; it defines the elements that will constitute what the different solutions attempt to respond to. This development of a given into a question, this transformation of a group of obstacles and difficulties into problems to which the diverse solutions will attempt to produce a response, this is what constitutes the point of problematization and the specific work of thought.

(Rabinow, 1984:389)

This is part of the project of this book, namely to look at how the discourse of ending AIDS is both seen as a solution to a problem and at the same time *becomes* its problematization; that is, the very term ending AIDS invokes certain solutions to the problem of AIDS which in themselves also are elements that should not be seen as the final solution to an issue, rather they are contingent, and are themselves open to critical analysis for the productive work they do. Furthermore, the book also responds to the question of what kind of obstacles does the discourse of ending AIDS aim at transforming, removing or controlling on the road to ending AIDS? How are the solutions proposed under such a regime also, in and of themselves, problematic? And finally, why did these and only these solutions emerge as possible solutions to the issue of HIV/AIDS?

It is also possible to read the importance of looking at the issue of ending AIDS as a problematization through the notion that a broad range of problematics arises in connection to the concept of uncertainty. Indeed, the very idea of ending AIDS should perhaps be framed within a certain notion of uncertainty. Many of the modalities for ending AIDS are predicated upon closing out or shutting down any notion of uncertainty ranging from the HIV test itself to epidemiological, disaggregated data mapping to statistics on how many are HIV positive, how many are on treatment and how many are virally suppressed. Yet uncertainty is never fully foreclosed in the discourse of ending AIDS. Where one set of (problematic) uncertainties seem to be dealt with, new uncertainties arise, such as will individuals adhere to their daily PrEP regimes or, with the rollout of PrEP, will condom usage decline and spur an increase in other sexually transmitted infections (STIs). Other new uncertainties might be linked to the development of HIV resistance or the impact of the new biomedical drugs that are being rolled out.

If we think of problems as creative responses to situations of uncertainty, then we have moved away from the circularities of subjection and resistance toward an account in which subjectivity is formed concerning horizons of difficulty, questioning and interrogation (Barnett, 2019). Part of the rationale for this book is to investigate how ending AIDS is both the answer to a problematization and, at the same time, is itself a form of problematization. The end of AIDS is thus the historical culmination at the present historical moment of a forty-year long process of problematizing the issue of HIV/AIDS.

There is, as such, a relationship between the ending of AIDS as an *object* to be ended as well as the *process* of problematizing this very end. Foucault highlights this connection between the object of problematization and the process of problematizing when he states that 'I think there is a relation between the thing that is problematized and the process of problematization. The problematization is an answer to a concrete situation which is real' (Michel Foucault, 2001:172). In saying this, Foucault also highlights that problematization goes beyond a mere critique of representation; that is, the representation of a problem, rather problematization is, in fact, a critique that concerns itself with practice and with the lived lives of people. This is a key point concerning the ending of AIDS as a historical narrative which this chapter concerns itself with and, on a more general level, is what this entire book is about. I am not arguing that the ending of AIDS as we see it in various textual documents are mere representations of a *real problem*; rather, I argue that these textual traces are in a very real way part and parcel of this *real situation* which Foucault states above. These documents that I will be analyzing and which are part and parcel of the ending of AIDS as a historical narrative are *creative responses to a particular concrete situation*, in this case, the HIV/AIDS epidemic. As Foucault states, 'a certain problematization is always a kind of creation; but a creation in the sense that, given a certain situation, you cannot infer that this kind of problematization will follow' (Michel Foucault, 2001:172). This takes us beyond an analysis which concerns itself only with representation; rather, the emphasis on the creative dimension of problematization underscores that the relationship under examination is not one merely of representation or even refraction of a situation in thought. Referencing Foucault again, we can state that

> Given a certain problematization, you can only understand why this kind of answer appears as a reply to some concrete and specific aspect of the world. There is a relation between thought and reality in the process of problematization. And that is the reason I think that it is possible to give an analysis of a specific problematization as the history of an answer – the original, specific and singular answer of thought – to a certain situation.
>
> (Michel Foucault, 2001:171)

This is also a premise that will be echoed in this book. The book is primarily not concerned with the various situations in which the end of AIDS is highlighted nor perhaps so much with the problem of HIV or AIDS; rather, its primary concern is how the figure of ending AIDS is a dynamic concept invoked by many in very friction-filled and creative ways. It is perhaps the thought of ending AIDS which this book is concerned with; however, this should not be taken to mean that there aren't real-life consequences to these thoughts. On the contrary, as this book will show the very problematization of ending AIDS indeed impacts people's lives in very profound and, in certain cases, very detrimental ways.

Following Clive Barnett, we could state that if we see the discourse of ending HIV as both the object of problematization and the active process of problematization then

> If we see problematizations as amplifications or intensifications of domains of engaged action, then the pressing analytical task is no longer viewed as one of critical disruption, but rather one of rearranging what is already

known, of seeking to 'make visible what is visible'. The notion of problematization might, in short, point toward a mode of descriptive analysis that helps to draw into view the significance of the difficulties and concerns that already animate people's actions. Rather than underwriting a model of critique in which it is presumed that people's subjectivities are readily available for re-making under the force of the revelatory exposure of contingency, elaborations of Foucault's notion of problematization invite us to give more credence to how aspects of people's subjectivity come to matter so strongly to them, and in turn to ask what price would have to be paid in the pursuit of transformation.

(Barnett, 2019)

In this very dense and useful quote from Barnett, we can link a few aspects directly to this book and its project of looking at what it means to 'end AIDS'; first of all, if the end of AIDS can be seen through the lens of problematization, then this book also aims at rearranging what we already take for granted about the end of AIDS, making the very term problematic. Secondly, it will draw into view the significance and the difficulties surrounding the end of AIDS as it figures in people's lives, in particular in this case, gay men and transgender women in the US, the UK and the Nordic context. Finally, it will also investigate what kind of price will be paid on the road to ending AIDS and ensuring an HIV-free generation; who will have to pay for this, at what cost, and in turn what kind of transformations will have to happen to ensure that this end comes about.

In looking at the end of AIDS as a specific form of problematization or problem, it of course also becomes clear that this rationale can be extended to all the aspects of the HIV epidemic. This also introduces a problem of limiting our analysis to a certain set of spaces wherein we can think problematically about the end of AIDS as I have elaborated upon above. The impact of the HIV epidemic and its reverberations can be felt well beyond the confines of it being an infectious disease as Paula Treichler and others have shown. The impact of the epidemic is just as much an epidemic of meaning and signifying practices as it is an infectious disease epidemic. This might be attributed to HIV being what Marcel Mauss called 'a total social fact' (Mauss, 2002). A total social fact is 'an activity that has implications throughout society, in the economic, legal, political and religious spheres' (Sedgwick & Edgar, 1999:64). In a more detailed wording of what a total social fact is, Mauss, states that

these phenomena are at once legal, economic, religious, aesthetic, morphological and so on. They are legal in that they concern individual and collective rights, organized and diffuse morality; they may be entirely obligatory, or subject simply to praise or disapproval. They are at once political and domestic, being of interest both to classes and to clans and families. They are religious; they concern true religion, animism, magic and diffuse religious mentality. They are economic […].

(Mauss, 2002)

In many ways, HIV has come to occupy a total social fact; that is, HIV is both a disease, an illness, a mediator caught in a moral, legal and social network of meaning-making, rendering it more than just a disease. It is implicated in a range of economic contexts, as well as religious discourses of redemption, blame, sin and morality. Finally, HIV entangles the individual with the collective and the private with the public.

To think problematically about the end of AIDS should not, however, be reduced to an analysis which just complicates what it might mean to end AIDS. Rather, it involves invoking a way of thinking about HIV, PrEP, epidemiological mapping and ARVs as specific problems that come to matter for people. As Barnett states, 'Foucault's account of problematization, which is the concern with how problems relate to the practical conduct of people's lives' (Barnett, 2019) is much richer than simply a manner of complicating the end of AIDS, as it were, in our case. Thus HIV and, by extension, epidemiological mapping, PrEP and ARVs become concrete instances wherein prescriptive norms take hold, practical actions are taken and people's lives are impacted, both positively and negatively, through these technologies intended to end AIDS. To analyze the end of AIDS as a form of problematization through these three modalities and in specific empirical spaces, as I will return to later in this chapter, means that 'the task of analysis becomes one of clarifying the conditions and situations to which problems are a response' (Barnett, 2019). In this sense, the analytical lens is moved onto how, for instance, PrEP as a response to the problem of HIV emerges as a specific form of response to HIV.

I want to paraphrase Michel Foucault as a way of providing a perhaps too bold a statement on the purpose of this book, but it is a statement I nevertheless want to make. Foucault stated in his piece *Fearless Speech* that

> For when I say that I am studying the 'problematization' of madness, crime or sexuality, it is not a way of denying the reality of such phenomena. On the contrary […] I think there is a relation between the thing that is problematized and the process of problematization. The problematization is an answer to a concrete situation which is real.
>
> (Michel Foucault, 2001:172)

In a somewhat similar fashion, I want to argue that this book is precisely about the problematization of the end of AIDS discourse; it is not an attempt to dismiss such an endeavor, rather it is to look at three concrete answers to the HIV epidemic in concrete situations and to critically analyze the end of AIDS as a specific form of problematizing HIV.

Paraphrasing Foucault again, we can state that "Given a certain problematization [ending AIDS], you can only understand why this kind of answer [PrEP, ARVs, epidemiological mapping, norms for sexual behavior, etc] appears as a reply to some concrete and specific aspect of the world [the

HIV epidemic]" (Michel Foucault, 2001:172). It is this that goes to the core of this book's rationale: the problematization of the signifying practices that have emerged in an era that proposes that the end of AIDS is within reach.

On method

This book is primarily based on a combination of images and texts. I have used a broad range of sources which I have treated as primary sources. I have focused mainly on sources found in science and medical journals, mass media news found online, articles published in gay and queer online news outlets, international organizations and their online documents and, finally, national strategies and reports. As Epstein stated in a slightly different setting (Epstein, 1996:355), my goal has been to analytically juxtapose contemporary records and sources in an effort to highlight how different social worlds comment upon, and make sense of, various strategies toward the end of AIDS. My analytical cue has been to assume that different social worlds and different actors and stakeholders engage differently in the construction of a narrative which subscribes to the notion that we can end AIDS. Bringing an eclectic set of sources and themes into proximity, as I have done in this book, allows us, I argue, to analyze how different stakeholders, actors and mediums construct, relate to and configure the end of AIDS narrative.

There is of course a caveat here: published stories only tell part of this story as Epstein noted in his work (Epstein, 1996:355). The same is true for my story in this book. In using textual sources and even images, we must also remember that these represent the end result of an oftentimes long and even contested process of becoming finished texts and images. 'Sometimes, in their linearity and smoothness, finished documents *conceal* the story' (Epstein, 1996: 355, original italics). Indeed, this is a pitfall of my own analysis; by using textual sources, even when they come from different sources and domains, the sources can only provide us with an overarching thematic structure of the end of AIDS. Yet, the claims made should be taken as part of a *narrative analysis* of the end of AIDS discourse – one that seeks to problematize *why, how and what effects* the end of AIDS narrative sets in motion as a signifying epidemic. In a way, I have also drawn on Michel Foucault's genealogical and archeological method in that I have tried to map the conditions of the different forms of knowledge that have come to bear upon the notion of an end to AIDS. Secondly, I have tried to show that the end of AIDS narrative is not the product of a linear nor homogenous discourse by drawing upon sources that show the shifts and discontinuities of the many different actors and their stakes in the end of AIDS narrative. By juxtaposing different sources, different themes, different knowledge regimes and different stakeholders, I have tried to be attentive to the contingent, the relational and the contested in the end of AIDS narrative.

Finally, I have tried to highlight the role of controversy and of what Foucault called 'subjugated knowledge'. The first is influenced by actor-network theory and the sociology of translation as found in the work of Bruno Latour (Latour, 1987; 1999). Here I have tried to highlight the many controversies and tensions that are present in the narrative of the end of AIDS. This also aligns with the term 'subjugated knowledge' which for Foucault encapsulates those knowledge claims made by actors and institutions which are not hegemonic, but rather, is knowledge that is often discounted, illegitimate or in opposition to the hegemonic, the privileged and the process of making knowledge hierarchies (Foucault, 2002). In doing this, I have tried to show a plethora of themes, claims, knowledge regimes and disciplines, all of which are part and parcel of the ways in which the end of AIDS is being communicated. More so, I have attended to parts of the visual economy of this signifying epidemic as well as utilizing the Internet as a prime mediator of knowledge, networking and of signification.

The goal of this book is to engage with what the end of AIDS signifies within certain domains of the social world – be that biomedical discourses, health promotions or strategies and reports. As such, this book tries to map and chart some of the ways in which the end of AIDS narrative is entangled with several different signifying practices, some of which might ultimately undermine the end of AIDS narrative itself.

Notes

1 See video; https://www.youtube.com/watch?v=_m4ks-H8Pww
2 See the campaign; http://hivstopswithme.org/
3 See the campaign; https://www.hivpreventionengland.org.uk/it-starts-with-me/
4 See UNAIDS fact sheet for 2017; http://www.unaids.org/en/resmyces/fact-sheet
5 See UNAIDS fact sheet; https://www.unaids.org/en/resources/fact-sheet
6 See Clive Barnett's article on the issue of problematization; https://nonsite.org/article/on-problematization

References

Anthony, S., & Fauci, M. (2019). HIV viral load and transmissibility of HIV infection undetectable equals untransmittable. Published by JAMA, Online First, January 10th, 2019.

Bacchi, C. (2012). Why study problematizations? Making politics visible. *Open Journal of Political Science*, *2*(1), 1.

Bacchi, C. (2015). The turn to problematization: Political implications of contrasting interpretive and poststructural adaptations. *Open Journal of Political Science*, *5*(1), 1–12. Scientific Research Publishing Inc.

Bacchi, C., & Goodwin, S. (2016). *Poststructural policy analysis: A guide to practice.* Berlin: Springer.

Barnett, C. (2019). On problematization. Elaborations on a theme in "late Foucault". *non .site.org, 6*. Retrieved from https://nonsite.org/article/on-problematization.

Benton, A., Sangaramoorthy, T., & Kalofonos, I. (2017). Temporality and positive living in the age of HIV/AIDS – A multi-sited ethnography. *Current Anthropology*, *58*(4), 454.

De Blasio, B. (2018). De Blasio Administration Announces Historic Low for New HIV Diagnoses, down 64 percent since reporting began in 2001. Retrieved from https://ww

w1.nyc.gov/office-of-the-mayor/news/578-18/de-blasio-administration-historic-low-new-hiv-diagnoses-down-64-percent-since.

Deleuze, G. (1994). *Difference and repetition*. New York, NY: Columbia University Press.

Eisinger, R. W., Dieffenbach, C. W., & Fauci, A. S. (2019). HIV viral load and transmissibility of HIV infection: Undetectable equals untransmittable. *JAMA, 321*(5), 451–452.

Farmer, P. (2006). *AIDS and accusation: Haiti and the geography of blame*. Berkeley, CA: University of California Press.

Fassin, D. (2007). *When bodies remember: Experiences and politics of AIDS in South Africa*, (Vol. 15). Berkeley, CA: University of California Press.

Foucault, M. (1984a). *The Foucault Reader* (Paul Rabinow, Ed.). (p. 173). New York, NY: Pantheon.

Foucault, M. (1984b). Polemics, politics, and problematizations. In Paul Rabinow (Ed.), *Foucault Reader* (pp. 381–390). New York, NY: Pantheon Books.

Foucault, M. (2001). *Fearless speech*. New York, NY: Semiotext (e).

Foucault, M. (2002). *The order of things: An archaeology of the human sciences*. Routledge, London: Psychology Press.

Foucault, M. (2012a). *The history of sexuality, vol. 2: The use of pleasure*. New York, NY: Vintage Book Company.

Foucault, M. (2012b). *The history of sexuality, vol. 3. The care of the self*. New York, NY: Vintage Book Company.

Foucault, M., Lotringer, S., & Hochroth, L. (2007). *The politics of truth*. Cambridge, MA: MIT Press.

Geuss, R. (2002). Genealogy as a critique. *European Journal of Philosophy, 10*(2), 209–215.

Hall, S. (1996). Cultural studies and its theoretical legacies. In David Morley and Kuan-Hsing Chen (Eds.), *Stuart Hall: Critical Dialogues in Cultural Studies* (pp. 262–275). London: Routledge.

Harris, T. G., Rabkin, M., & El-Sadr, W. M. (2018). Achieving the fourth 90: healthy aging for people living with HIV. *AIDS (London, England), 32*(12), 1563.

HIV.Gov. (2019). What is 'ending the HIV epidemic: A plan for America'? Retrieved from https://www.hiv.gov/federal-response/ending-the-hiv-epidemic/overview.

Kenworthy, N., Thomann, M., & Parker, R. (2018a). Critical perspectives on the 'end of AIDS'. *Global Public Health, 13*(8), 1–3.

Kenworthy, N., Thomann, M., & Parker, R. (2018b). From a global crisis to the 'end of AIDS': New epidemics of signification. *Global Public Health, 13*(8), 960–971.

Kippax, S., & Stephenson, N. (2016). *Socializing the biomedical turn in HIV prevention*. London, New York, NY: Anthem Press.

Koopman, C. (2011). Foucault across the disciplines: Introductory notes on contingency in critical inquiry. *History of the Human Sciences, 24*(4), 1–12.

Mauss, M. (2002). *The gift: The form and reason for exchange in archaic societies*. London, New York, NY: Routledge.

Miller, P., & Rose, N. (2008). *Governing the present: Administering economic, social and personal life*. Cambridge: Polity.

Miller, P., & Rose, N. (2017). Political power beyond the state: Problematics of government. In Peter Fitzpatrick (Ed.), *Foucault & Law* (pp. 191–224). London, New York, NY: Routledge.

New York City Department of Public Health. (2020). *Prevent HIV and other STIs*. Retrieved from https://www1.nyc.gov/site/doh/health/health-topics/playsure.page.

Nguyen, V.-K. (2010). *The republic of therapy: Triage and sovereignty in West Africa's Time of AIDS*. Durham, NC: Duke University Press.

Nguyen, V.-K., O'Malley, J., & Pirkle, C. M. (2011). Remedicalizing an epidemic: From HIV treatment as prevention to HIV treatment is prevention. *AIDS, 25*(11), 1435.

PEPFAR. (2017). Strategy for accelerating HIV/AIDS epidemic control (2017–2020). Retrieved from https://www.state.gov/wp-content/uploads/2019/08/PEPFAR-Strategy-for-Accelerating-HIVAIDS-Epidemic-Control-2017-2020.pdf.

Rabinow, P. (1984). Polemics, politics, and problematizations. An interview with Michel Foucault. *The Foucault Reader*, 380–390.

Race, K. (2017). *The gay science: Intimate experiments with the problem of HIV*. London, New York, NY: Routledge.

Sedgwick, P., & Edgar, A. (1999). *Key concepts in cultural theory*. London, New York, NY: Routledge.

Shore, C., & Wright, S. (2015). Governing by numbers: Audit culture, rankings and the new world order. *Social Anthropology, 23*(1), 22–28.

Sidibé, M., Loures, L., & Samb, B. (2016). The UNAIDS 90–90–90 target: A clear choice for ending AIDS and for sustainable health and development. *Journal of the International AIDS Society, 19*(1), 21133.

Treichler, P. A. (1999). *How to have theory in an epidemic: Cultural Chronicles of AIDS*. Durham, NC: Duke University Press.

Trickey, A., May, M. T., Vehreschild, J.-J., Obel, N., Gill, M. J., Crane, H. M. ... Cazanave, C. (2017). Survival of HIV-positive patients starting antiretroviral therapy between 1996 and 2013: A collaborative analysis of cohort studies. *The Lancet HIV, 4*(8), e349–e356.

UN. (2015). *RES/70/1. Transforming our world: The 2030 agenda for sustainable development* (p. 25). New York, NY: Seventieth United Nations General Assembly.

UNAIDS. (2014a). 90-90-90: An ambitious treatment target to help end the AIDS epidemic. Geneva: UNAIDS.

UNAIDS. (2014b). AIDS 2014: Galvanizing a movement for ending the AIDS epidemic by 2030.

UNAIDS. (2016). Political declaration on HIV and AIDS: On the fast-track to accelerate the fight against HIV and to end the AIDS epidemic by 2030. New York, NY: United Nations.

UNAIDS. (2018a). Miles to go—Closing gaps, breaking barriers, righting injustices. 268.

UNAIDS. (2018b). Progress report on the global plan. *UNAIDS 2015*.

UNAIDS. (2019). Global HIV & AIDS statistics — 2019 Fact sheet. Retrieved from https ://www.unaids.org/en/resources/fact-sheet.

Warner, M. (2002). *Publics and counterpublic*. New York, NY: Zone Books.

2 A short history toward the end of AIDS

The current drive to end AIDS did not emerge *ex nihlo*. Establishing monikers such as 'ending AIDS by 2030' or 'ensuring an HIV-free generation' has taken a tremendous amount of work across diverse sectors, national boundaries, communities and agencies. This chapter is less a deep analysis of the history of the biomedicalization of the HIV epidemic than it is a genealogy of the emergence of the UNAIDS 90-90-90 targets and the subsequent push to end AIDS. It is a necessary chapter to familiarize the reader with the various biomedical turns that have happened within the HIV epidemic and to make it contextually clearer why the very phrase 'ending AIDS' could emerge when it emerged. Lukas Engelmann, in his in-depth study of the mapping of the AIDS epidemic, states that 'the now-normalized idea that our epoch has somehow resolved the crisis of AIDS seems in need of a convincing narrative in which the notion of an *old* AIDS is successfully separated from the time of the *new* AIDS' (Engelmann, 2018). This chapter delineates some of the temporal dimensions of the AIDS epidemic in just this fashion. Stated differently, it delineates some key moments that have led to the formation of a narrative of 'post-crisis' and the end of AIDS, while also stressing that any easy periodization of the HIV/AIDS epidemic into a 'crisis' and a 'post-crisis' period or a 'HAART/ARV' era and a 'pre-ARV' era is a dangerous linear periodization which fails to recognize the many millions who do not have access to ARVs and the many people who do still die from AIDS-related illnesses or suffer under the stigma of HIV.

From treatment and prevention to treatment as prevention: the second wave of pharamaceuticalization and the possibility of an 'HIV-free generation'

Since the introduction of antiretroviral treatment (ARV) for HIV, the push for treatment access has been a dominant focus. This was for the longest time balanced with a need for *preventive* measures – mainly condom usage, but also behavioral changes, such as limiting the number of sexual partners and offering clean needle programs for people who inject drugs. As such, there was a split between treatment and prevention. However, in recent years, this divide has become porous through the paradigm of 'treatment as prevention'.

While the ARV era was ushered in after the FDA authorized the first pro-tease inhibitor in 1995, it wasn't until the HPTN 052 trial in 2011 (M. S. Cohen, McCauley, & Gamble, 2012) that the link between ARV regimes, early initiation of treatment and prevention was formed. The HPTN trial showed that

> early initiation of antiretroviral therapy (ART) for the HIV-positive partner reduced cases of onward transmission to the HIV-negative partner by 96% compared to delayed treatment. Early treatment also resulted in 41% fewer adverse health events for the person living with HIV compared to those not receiving treatment until their CD4 count fell to 200–250 copies per mm.
>
> (Cohen et al., 2011)

This finding was seen as 'a game-changer' and was even named 'breakthrough of the year' in the journal Science (J. Cohen, 2011b). The HPTN 052 trial proved two key issues: that people who started treatment earlier had less risk of developing 'severe, category 4 events' (M. S. Cohen et al., 2011) which meant that people who started ART sooner were less likely to fall ill and would thus be more healthy; and, that amongst couples wherein one was HIV-positive and the other was HIV-negative, viral load suppression meant that the positive partner was unable to transmit HIV to the negative partner. The results of the HPTN 052 trial were confirmed by the 2014 PARTNER trial (Rodger et al., 2016) in which a total of 58,000 sex acts without condoms were observed and zero new HIV infections occurred. These two studies, alongside mounting evidence that the lowering of viral loads to so-called 'undetectable levels' led to uninfectious-ness, heralded the treatment as a prevention paradigm which is currently the hegemonic model for public health prevention in terms of stopping onward HIV infections.

Anthony Fauci, the head of the US National Institute of Allergy and Infectious Diseases, and a looming authority within the field of HIV/AIDS even went on record after the data of the HPTN 052 results came out and stated, 'The idea of the tension between treatment and prevention, we should just forget about it and just put it behind us because treatment is prevention' (J. Cohen, 2011b:1628). The HPTN 052 trial was seen as a revolution and a true game-changer of the HIV epidemic in that

> The HPTN 052 results and other recent successes have raised hopes that com-bining such interventions can now end AIDS epidemics in entire countries, if not the world. ARVs are not a vaccine: People must take them for decades, which is difficult to do and costly.
>
> (J. Cohen, 2011b:1628)

Yet the HPTN 052 trial was seen as a push for *more* ARVs not only for their prop-erties in *treating* HIV, but also for their *preventive* effects.

Gone were so many of the objections, uncertainties and debates that had plagued the early ARV discussions described in the work of Steven Epstein

(Epstein, 1996). In fact, as Julio Montaner, a prominent HIV researcher from Canada stated, 'Clinicians and policymakers are always asking for the ultimate evidence, HPTN 052 was the unequivocal piece of the puzzle to close any doubts' (J. Cohen, 2011b:1628). In Montaner and Fauci's words, treatment as prevention (TasP) was indeed a game-changer, one that would herald the 'end of AIDS' and which would also spur then President of the United States, Barack Obama, to declare a policy platform which would ensure an 'AIDS-free generation' (J. Cohen, 2011a:1338). TasP, in short, has been nothing but a remarkable invention within HIV prevention.

While TasP manifested itself once and for all after the release of the HPTN 052 results, the idea of TasP had been around for some time before the trial. As Guillaume Lachenal states, 'TasP began as an exercise in epidemiological modeling' which tried to answer the question of 'Knowing that antiretroviral therapy drastically reduces HIV transmission, what population-level effect would result from screening and immediately treating all HIV-infected individuals?' (Lachenal, 2013:70). As a form of problematization, this question was given an 'answer' by WHO expert, Reuben Granich, who stated in an article from 2009 that 'universal voluntary HIV testing once a year of all people older than 15 years, combined with immediate ART after diagnosis, could bring about a phase change in the nature of the epidemic' (R. M. Granich, Gilks, Dye, De Cock, & Williams, 2009:54). Furthermore, Granich et al. stated that

> Although other prevention interventions, alone or in combination, could substantially reduce HIV incidence, our model suggests that only universal voluntary HIV testing and immediate initiation of ART could reduce transmission to the point at which elimination might be feasible by 2020 for a generalized epidemic.
>
> (R. M. Granich et al., 2009:54)

Granich et al. and their modeling study stipulated that implementing their universal and voluntary testing regime as well as the immediate start-up of ARVs would, by 2050, lead to HIV infection rates at very low and manageable levels (R. M. Granich et al., 2009:55). While the statement itself might not be exceptionally different from other biomedical 'answers' about how to bring about the elimination of the HIV epidemic, it is the use of data modeling as *the only* way to reach an end that interests me here.

Marsha Rosengarten and Mike Michael have written convincingly on the performative function of modeling and how modeling on PrEP studies creates a notion of a 'stable product' in the case of PrEP (Michael & Rosengarten, 2013; Rosengarten & Michael, 2009). My point is that part of the emergence of the notion that treatment is prevention and that this could lead to the elimination and end of HIV rests on the performative aspect of data modeling such as Granich's study. Paraphrasing Michael and Rosengarten's 'stability can be enacted through the added technology of statistical modeling. While such modeling functions as a valuable predictor, here it serves as a type of exemplar of the work of expectation'

(Rosengarten & Michael, 2009:1053): while the introduction of ARVs had shown in clinical settings that onward transmission was limited by suppression of viral load, modeling studies such as Granich's provided a performative exemplar that played on and further heightened the expectation that, indeed, ARV as TasP had the potential to end the HIV epidemic. This of course rested upon, as Granich et al. note, mass testing and subsequent start-up of ARVs.

However, the study also mentioned the perceived weaknesses of the model which was the need for better data (R. M. Granich et al., 2009:54) on a broad range of issues, such as 'the acceptability and uptake of universal voluntary HIV testing, the infectiousness of people receiving ART, adherence, behavior change after starting ART and rates of emergence of resistance' (R. M. Granich et al., 2009:54). Of note here is, of course, that most of these 'weaknesses' of the study are highly *personalized*. Most of these issues relate to the individual subject and not to the broader social drivers of the HIV epidemic nor to the health care systems that are expected to carry out mass HIV testing and start-up of ARVs. In this regard, a reading in 'bad faith' would perhaps read Granich's study as placing the problem of ending HIV not on the model, or the structural issues of the HIV epidemic, but rather on the individual.

Many of these 'weak data points', as Granich et al. might have called them, are highly predicated upon social, cultural and economic factors. For instance, acceptability and uptake are often predicated upon cultural norms for health behavior, while talking about sex and issues of intimacy depend upon social norms, and uptake has as much to do with economic access to treatment as it has to do with robust health care systems and the trust that exists between the population and the health care authorities (Angotti, 2012; Luginaah, Yiridoe, & Taabazuing, 2005; MacPhail, Pettifor, Coates, & Rees, 2008). Adherence is also another issue in which models fail; adherence has, for a long time, been a thorny issue in both HIV prevention and in other health care settings, such as psychiatry, diabetes treatment and the monitoring and treatment of high blood pressure. In a way, many of these issues are issues that 'escape datafication'; that is, the quantification and mathematical modeling of many of these data points, such as the ones that Granich used, are difficult to translate from lived lives to models. Once again paraphrasing Michael and Rosengarten, it is important to note that the use of modeling studies such as Granich's study enacts mass HIV testing and subsequent start-up of ARVs as a form of *stable intervention* and enacts it as a distinct entity amongst other HIV preventive initiatives (Rosengarten & Michael, 2009:1053). This is important, for, even with its many weaknesses, the data model that Granich's study produced showed that 'TasP promised to overcome unending hesitations about whether to prioritize treatment or prevention in resource-limited settings: it would do both' (Lachenal, 2013:70). In the case of TasP, Granich's model can be seen as part of the push for a biomedical solution to the problem of HIV. While it wasn't until the HPTN 052 trial that TasP finally emerged as a public health care regime aimed at ending AIDS, data models, such as Granich's, did play a part in 'stabilizing' the idea of mass treatment as not just treatment, but rather as *prevention* that was crucial to reach the end of AIDS. However, while the concept of treatment as prevention has become a major pillar within the quest to end AIDS, and while it has proved to provide high rates of effective HIV prevention, some issues have come up in terms of how the treatment as prevention regime has been rolled out, and how it has been implemented.

Vinh-Kim Nguyen noted, in 2011, that while

> increased investment in treatment is welcomed, it is profoundly disturbing that prevention remains grossly underfunded even as treatment budgets explode. Nowhere are the dangers of this remedicalization clearer than in the case of 'treatment-as-prevention' (TASP), widely trumpeted as a 'game-changer' and a 'paradigm shift' in the battle against HIV/AIDS.
>
> (Nguyen, O'Malley, & Pirkle, 2011:291)

For Nguyen et al., the TasP paradigm was seen as a much-welcomed addition to the quest to end AIDS, yet they also mention at least three potential problems with the treatment as prevention paradigm. First of all, they state that the framing of TasP as a sort of 'magic bullet' to end AIDS has some serious flaws. 'For TASP to work as a prevention strategy, at least 75% of HIV-positive individuals must be diagnosed and treated' (Nguyen et al., 2011:291). The issue that Nguyen et al. has with this part of the discourse around TasP is that it is highly unlikely that we will achieve these numbers if we do not pay 'serious attention to the social inequalities and stigmatization that already determine vulnerability to acquiring HIV and accessibility of diagnosis and treatment' (Nguyen et al., 2011:291). TasP should be seen in relation to and against a backdrop that 'should be viewed appropriately as a humane response to the suffering brought on by infection with prevention possibilities. It is not a substitute for the removal of the vulnerabilities that place people at risk of infection in the first place' (Nguyen et al., 2011:291). The second point they note in their paper is that while TasP is welcomed as a supplement on the road to achieving an HIV-free generation, the shift in focus from an HIV paradigm based on 'rights here, right now' to a focus on biomedical interventions, such as TasP, can lead to a foreclosing of a 'lively and vigorous debate on their [TasP] effectiveness and their implications' (Nguyen et al., 2011:291). The fear here is that the push for treatment as prevention in the name of ending AIDS will diminish, undermine and ultimately push to the side the important work still left in ensuring that vulnerable people have the right to lead long and healthy lives and are guaranteed access to treatment, testing and harm reduction initiatives and other socio-economic programs meant to ensure high quality of life, good health and wellbeing.

Finally, the third issue that Nguyen et al. warn us about in terms of the TasP regime lies in the following postulate:

> in the rush to paradigm shift, game-change, roll out, and scale up yet a new set of acronyms and standardized interventions, local epidemiological, political, and socio-historical context is once again being ignored, surely only to resurface later as 'culture' once much-heralded interventions fail to deliver.

> Holding out for a magic bullet – unlikely to ever come – diminishes interest in the hard, messy work required to enable social change and address the social inequalities and structural violence that drive this epidemic. Biomedical interventions are unlikely to live up to their promise if social determinants of access to prevention and treatment are not addressed.
>
> (Nguyen et al., 2011:291)

As we see in the formulations from Nguyen et al. here, the heralding of TasP as a sort of magic bullet to end AIDS should be taken with a grain of salt. It is not so much the TasP regime nor its scale-up that is at issue. Rather, it is the potential effects that it produces, such as an increased focus on biomedical interventions to the detriment of focus on larger structural issues as well as the potential pitfalls of implementing TasP interventions that ignore localized dynamics, cultural sensibilities and local economic and political contexts. In the end, Nguyen and his co-authors point to issues that have a long history in scholarship on the HIV epidemic, made manifest in the scholarship of medical doctor and anthropologist Paul Farmer in his work on the structural violence embedded within the HIV epidemic and the need to address issues such as poverty, stigma and legal prosecution of people living with HIV, minorities and lack of access to health care (Farmer, 2004, 2006).

However, TasP and the modeling study which laid the foundation for it were crucial to the notion that 'we' could globally end AIDS through a new paradigm for prevention which went through the route of 'test, treat and retain'. This set the stage for what I have called the 'synchronization of the end of AIDS' which is what I will dedicate the next section of this chapter too.

Role of targets and indicators: the logic behind the End of AIDS

In the period before what is now known as the 'ARV era', the HIV epidemic was often talked about as a global crisis. The HIV/AIDS epidemic is the only epidemic to have been taken up in the UN Security Council two times, with two subsequent UN resolutions – Res. 1983 and Res. 1308. In both cases, the HIV/AIDS epidemic was framed as a crisis of global proportions such as in Res. 1308, where the Security Council stated: 'the HIV/AIDS pandemic, if unchecked, may pose a risk to stability and security' (UNAIDS, 2000). This was reiterated in Res.1983, when the Security Council made the statement that 'HIV poses one of the most formidable challenges to the development, progress and stability of societies and requires an exceptional and comprehensive global response' (UNAIDS, 2011). Kenworthy et al. state that

> if the decade following the first Durban AIDS Conference in 2000 was marked by discourses about an epidemic 'out of control' and a politics of emergency that justified exceptional activism and action, the decade of AIDS responses beginning in 2010 has been distinctly framed by declarations that an AIDS-free generation is within our grasp.
>
> (N. Kenworthy, Thomann, & Parker, 2018b:960)

In framing the history of the HIV/AIDS epidemic in this fashion, Kenworthy et al. not only point out the recent shift in the framing of the HIV epidemic but also highlight the *periodization* of the epidemic.

While the introduction of the so-called 'ARV era' ushered in what AVERT claims 'led to a period of optimism',[1] the HIV epidemic was by the late 1990s and early 2000s framed as a 'global crisis' and, in particular, an African crisis (Piot, 2003; Sibanda, 2000). As reported by the *New Scientist* in November of 2003, the UN sounded the alarms and reported that 2003 had 'the highest ever number of new HIV infections and deaths around the world' (Battacharya, 2003). Then UNAIDS Executive Director Peter Piot, stated in the same article that 'It is quite clear that our current global efforts remain entirely inadequate for an epidemic that is continuing to spiral out of control' (Battacharya, 2003). Jack Chow, assistant director-general for HIV/AIDS, TB and malaria at the World Health Organization, added that 'In two short decades HIV/AIDS has tragically become the premier disease of mass destruction' (Battacharya, 2003). By turning our attention to the situation back in the early 2000s, we also can see that while the rollout ARV drugs and a renewed optimism linked to the effect of these drugs which, as we know, were already rolled out in 1995, the word crisis and 'an epidemic out of control' still struck a chord in the global health community in the early 2000s.

Returning to some of the background discourses which shifted this temporal focus from crisis to ending AIDS, we should note that a few years after 2003 the financial crisis of 2007–2008 heralded a shift in funding which also spurred on the need for a new way of conceptualizing the HIV epidemic. Kenworthy et al. state that 'as a result of the financial crisis, a series of important donor withdrawals marked the beginning of a shift from "scale-up" to "scale-down" that still is visible today' (N. Kenworthy et al., 2018b:962) wherein donors are asking recipients to do more with less and 'optimize' their HIV treatment and prevention programs. This also meant that a new discourse of sustainability, accountability and country ownership, as well as the much talked about paradigm of transitioning from donor funding to domestic funding, took form as a way for donor countries to avoid long-term treatment commitments and resource-intensive programs (Engebretsen, Heggen, Das, Farmer, & Ottersen, 2016; Engebretsen, Heggen, & Ottersen, 2017; N. Kenworthy et al., 2018b). Following the scale-down and the paradigm of doing more with less, various national agencies and donor organizations shifted their funding strategies from general population and treatment scale-ups onto new targets such as 'key populations' and investments in biomedical prevention technologies and techniques. This can be seen in the shift of PEPFAR's latest sets of strategy plans (PEPFAR, 2018, 2017, 2016) wherein a shift toward a focus on key populations has become marked and rhetorically built upon the notion of 'partnership' and country ownership between PEPFAR and recipient countries.

The scale-down focus and cost-effectiveness focus that followed in the wake of the financial crisis was not limited to a reorientation in terms of donor–recipient relationships and their funding strategies; it also came at a time when the so-called 'AIDS backlash' was in full effect as both Kenworthy et al. and Nattrass and Gonsalves note (N. Kenworthy et al., 2018b; Nattrass & Gonsalves, 2009, 2010). This backlash implied emerging concern that HIV-specific funding and programs overshadowed other public health programs with higher mortality rates and a higher general prevalence, in particular in the global North. The AIDS backlash also resulted in growing concerns that rather than disease-specific approaches to HIV/AIDS, funding should be focused on strengthening health care systems in general (Nattrass, 2014; Nattrass & Gonsalves, 2009, 2010). Health system strengthening did gain a lot of traction and many in the global HIV industry saw this as a way of defending their new scale-down funding streams (Hafner & Shiffman, 2012). Crucial for our purposes in this chapter is the emergence of what can perhaps be called the 'prototype template' for the ending AIDS narrative which also signaled a renewed focus on HIV-specific funding as well as a new way of synchronizing the HIV/AIDS efforts.

In 2010, UNAIDS launched its *Getting to Zero: 2011–2016 Strategy* (UNAIDS, 2010). The strategy was built on the goals of zero new infections, zero AIDS-related deaths and zero discrimination (UNAIDS, 2010:7). The strategy was enshrined and adopted in 2011 by the UN General Assembly in its UNGASS declaration which stated that by 2015, fifty percent of the getting to zero goals would be reached (N. Kenworthy et al., 2018b:963). In 2014, UNAIDS launched its 'Fast Track' platform which built on the 90-90-90 targets and explicitly stated that the 'end of AIDS' was not only a possibility but could become a reality if the global community 'synchronized' their efforts according to the time frame of the 90-90-90 targets (which was 2020) and followed the initiatives proposed by the 90-90-90 strategy (UNAIDS, 2014). This was officially adopted in June of 2016 when the fast track platform was adopted within the *Political Declaration on HIV and AIDS: On the Fast Track to Accelerate the Fight against HIV and to Ending the AIDS Epidemic by 2030* (UNAIDS, 2016). This was predicated upon both evidence-based research in clinical settings and data modeling of epidemiological data. As such, there has been an immense drive to roll out various HIV treatment and prevention efforts to reach the 90-90-90 targets. This push is connected to recent developments in HIV biomedical prevention/treatment technologies which have been heralded as 'the beginning of the end of AIDS' (J. Cohen, 2011b). Several international stakeholders subscribe to the idea that the end of AIDS is not only a possibility, but is also an imminent event (Sidibé, Loures, & Samb, 2016; UNAIDS, 2014).

Before proceeding, it might be worth noting a key aspect of the slogan of 'ending AIDS', as this moniker can at times present some confusion. While the slogan itself seems to indicate a literal 'end to AIDS', it is important to keep in mind that the strategy as it is embodied in the 90-90-90 targets is *not* a campaign to globally eradicate HIV. While many of the currently circulating slogans that play on notions of 'ending AIDS' or as NYC Mayor Bill de Blasio stated, 'eradicating the epidemic', the fact of the matter is that the 90-90-90 targets aim at *controlling* the epidemic.

In epidemiological terms, there is a crucial difference to be made here. Epidemiological control is when transmission rates are reduced to what the WHO and the CDC notes are a 'reduction of disease incidence, prevalence, morbidity or mortality to a locally acceptable level as a result of deliberate efforts. Continued intervention is required to sustain control' (WHO, 2006). Elimination, on the other hand, implies 'the interruption of local transmission (that is, reducing the rate of malaria cases to zero) of a specified pathogen or parasite in a defined geographic area. Continued measures are required to prevent the re-establishment of transmission'. Finally, eradication means 'permanent reduction to zero of the worldwide incidence of infection caused by a specific agent as a result of deliberate efforts; intervention measures are no longer needed' (CDC, 1999). The 90-90-90 targets subsequently are aimed at achieving epidemic control and not as the popular slogan goes, 'an end to AIDS' such as elimination or eradication. Indeed, without a cure or a vaccine, the eradication of HIV is a distant goal, one that no single nation has yet to achieve. As Sara Davis notes, the WHO does not even have a process to validate that a country has eliminated HIV, a process they have for most other infectious diseases and pathogens (Davis, 2020). As such, the end of AIDS seems to be more about the *control* of HIV. In this book, I examine what sorts of control mechanisms have been developed recently as well as what they signify. Indeed, if ending AIDS is about control more than it is about elimination or eradication, what does this imply for the many signifying practices that emerge in this context?

Following these developments, by 2014 most donor agencies began to endorse and promote this new drive to end AIDS through first the fast track platform and then the 90-90-90 targets. The Global Fund, PEPFAR and USAID issued statements that now heralded the end of AIDS through the 90-90-90 targets; even in the private sector this became the new discourse toward which HIV/AIDS programs were pivoting (N. Kenworthy et al., 2018b:964). With the formation of the UN SDGs, the drive toward a temporal end date for AIDS seemed to be firmly set in place. These developments can not be seen as being purely developed within a frame of economy and political commitments; rather we should keep in mind the developments of various new biomedical technologies of treatment and prevention, which several scholars have pointed out were key in enabling the end of AIDS narrative to take hold (N. Kenworthy, Thomann, & Parker, 2018a; N. Kenworthy et al., 2018b; N.J. Kenworthy & Parker, 2014; Leclerc-Madlala, Broomhall, & Fieno, 2018; Sangaramoorthy, 2018).

What is of note for me in this chapter, though, is how the 90-90-90 targets not only have been developed in the wake of specific economic structures of funding and a historical narrative which has seen the HIV/AIDS epidemic go from one of crisis to a post-crisis climate, but also how this new temporal order within the global efforts to 'end AIDS' is made possible by recourse to the tools of biomedicalization and new technology purporting to be able to end AIDS. Kenworthy et al. state that

> while the concept of ending the epidemic began to be floated by global AIDS administrators as early as 2010, it then took roughly five years of sloganeering and issuing lower level UN documents to gradually get to the point

where it would become an official policy declaration adopted by the General Assembly.

(N. Kenworthy et al., 2018b:963)

While I agree with this analysis of the process leading up to the adaptation of the 90-90-90 targets and the subsequent 'end of AIDS' narrative, I think it also points us toward the vast apparatus of synchronization that went into effect through this process.

With the introduction of the 90-90-90 targets, certain 'lines of sights', as Beer notes, were emerging (Beer, 2016). Targets and metrics and the setting of these are often contested and subject to conflicting values in terms of what targets are most useful, which indicators should be used, etc. In relation to this, targets when finalized, seem to create lines of sight or focal points that are highlighted as being important. In the 90-90-90 targets, perhaps the most crucial step was to focus on the first 90 – that is, making sure that 90 percent of all people living with HIV know their HIV status. As Sara Davis notes, this also highlights the need for global and national health authorities to make an accurate estimate on the baseline number of people living with HIV in their countries and then making sure that 90 percent of these take an HIV test to know their status (Davis, 2020). While focusing on HIV testing has long been a core pillar in HIV prevention, the new 90-90-90 targets seem to indeed be contingent upon this initial step to be successful for the entire cascade to be successful. Massive HIV testing was indeed the bedrock upon which the initial 90-90-90 data model was based (Granich, Williams, Montaner, & Zuniga, 2017; Granich et al., 2009). As such, controlling the HIV epidemic through the 90-90-90 targets hinges, it seems, on massive HIV testing efforts. However, this is rendered less effective if the estimates are made on how many people live with HIV in a given country. Once again, we see that the end of AIDS is increasingly contingent and entangled with numerical targets, statistical data and subsequent indicator settings.

90-90-90: Three metrics, one goal, many gaps and issues

On October 25, 2014, then UNAIDS Executive Director Michel Sidibé, took to the stage in Hanoi at a UNAIDS summit and stated that

> This bold new set of targets, 90-90-90, will do more than reduce new HIV infections and AIDS-related deaths. It will be a transformative agenda for reaching people who are left behind [...] 90-90-90 is our path to victory. It is our path to the end of this epidemic worldwide. When we talk about ending AIDS, we mean that by 2030, HIV and AIDS will no longer threaten human life. Of course, there will be new cases of HIV, but the virus will no longer be a public health danger.

(Sidibe, 2014)

The above quote, from former UNAIDS Executive Director Michel Sidibé from the launch of the 90-90-90 targets in 2014, points to perhaps the most important pillar in the work toward the end of AIDS, that is, the rollout and scale-up of global 'test, treat and retain' efforts operationalized and quantified through the metrics of 90-90-90. The very phrasing that the 90-90-90 targets are the path to victory and the end of the HIV epidemic is telling for how a set of metrics becomes a form of governing or directing efforts to end AIDS. This also set into motion a broad push amongst nations and cities to be the first to reach these targets. In response to this, UNAIDS releases data on the progress toward the 90-90-90 targets and which countries have either reached them, are close to reaching them or are 'lagging behind'. For instance, three years later, in 2017, UNAIDS stated that seven countries had achieved the 90-90-90. These were Botswana, Cambodia, Denmark, Iceland, Singapore, Sweden and the United Kingdom (UNAIDS, 2017a:31). In connection to the report *Ending AIDS: Progress toward the 90-90-90 targets* (UNAIDS, 2017a), then Executive Director Michel Sidibe stated that

> When I launched the 90–90–90 targets three years ago, many people thought they were impossible to reach. Today, the story is very different. Families, communities, cities and countries have witnessed a transformation, with access to HIV treatment accelerating in the past three years. A record 19.5 million people are accessing antiretroviral therapy, and, for the first time, more than half of all people living with HIV are on treatment [...] Global solidarity and shared responsibility have driven the success we have achieved so far. This must be sustained [...] I remain optimistic. This report demonstrates the power of the 90–90–90 targets and what can be achieved in a short time.
>
> (UNAIDS, 2017a:6)

Clearly, in both 2014 and 2017, the UNAIDS and the world saw the potential in the 90-90-90 targets as a way of 'ending AIDS'. Yet the 90-90-90 targets also pose a series of problems, one of which is temporal. In working with these targets, one might get the sense that the end of AIDS will come when we have reached the 90-90-90 targets. The slogan, as well as the subsequent target-setting, might give us the impression that the end of AIDS is some sort of final event, or that once the targets have been reached the end has come. However, since the 90-90-90 targets are about epidemic control, continual work is needed to maintain the numbers. The slogan of ending AIDS and the 90-90-90 targets with their set deadlines belies the fact that ending AIDS through these targets is not a static or 'one-off' event. Without a vaccine or a cure, the end of AIDS will need to be *maintained*, and this will require continual monitoring, progress reporting and, most of all, continual engagement from all stakeholders.

This aspect can be seen as Sara Davis shows us, when in 2019, UNAIDS launched its *Miles to Go* report (UNAIDS, 2018a). This time, in 2019, updated data showed that now the list of 'successes' was reduced to six, and, while Botswana and the UK were still on the list, the others from the 2016 list had fallen out (Davis, 2020). They, in turn, had been replaced by Eswatini, Namibia and the Netherlands (UNAIDS, 2018a:72). The point I want to raise here is that while the end of AIDS has come to signify a new form of thinking about the HIV epidemic, the notion that there will be an 'event' that is the end of AIDS, a sort of punctuation mark of the HIV epidemic, should be tempered by a realization that epidemic control is not a result, but indeed a state of continually maintaining control. The concept of control can perhaps be metaphorically extended to epidemic control, which is about controlling the spread of HIV through various forms of HIV surveillance. Moreover, it is also about *self-control*. In many of the HIV health promotions that I have analyzed in the chapters to come, epidemic control is linked to controlling one's sexual health through various forms of self-control. As such, ending AIDS through the 90-90-90 targets and the notion of epidemic control, is a continual process of maintaining control, both at the level of the nation-state and at the level of the individual.

People and places: focusing on the 'right places and the right people'

Ending AIDS and the logic behind it was, as we have seen, born at the intersection of novel biomedical pharmaceuticals, advanced epidemiological modeling studies, political tensions between donor and recipient countries and a new economic reality in the wake of the financial crisis. With declining global funds dedicated to the HIV/AIDS efforts, donor countries and organizations started to talk more about the need for 'strategic' interventions that would 'maximize impact'. This language was adopted by PEPFAR, in particular through their renewed plan to focus on 13 countries which are near reaching 'epidemic control' (PEPFAR, 2018). PEPFAR has programs in 50 countries, yet with its new strategy of focusing on a select group of 13 countries that are close to achieving epidemic control, efforts are being redirected to these 13 countries. The 13 countries are Botswana, Côte d'Ivoire, Haiti, Kenya, Lesotho, Malawi, Namibia, Rwanda, Swaziland, Tanzania, Uganda, Zambia and Zimbabwe. Of note is the fact that all of them are in sub-Saharan African countries signaling what PEPFAR has called their 'transitioning out' of many low-prevalence and middle-income countries in both Eastern Europe, Central Asia, Asia, Latin America and the Caribbean. It also demonstrates other problematic aspects of the new focus on strategic interventions aimed at maximizing impact in the name of ending AIDS.

In the aftermath of the announcement that PEPFAR would shift its focus onto these 13 countries, renowned online media outlet, Devex, ran a series of articles on the implications of this shift. In the series, it was noted that 'some nonpriority countries have seen funds shrink' and that 'dramatic cuts to two priority countries during the current funding round, Tanzania and Kenya, took civil society organizations by surprise' (Green, 2019). Furthermore, it was noted that 'with these cuts, PEPFAR is intensifying its message that if a country is not making progress toward specific targets, either for programmatic or policy reasons, then the money will go elsewhere' (Green, 2019). Part of this was linked to how PEPFAR expected and expects recipient countries to 'do their part', that is, domestic funding dedicated to the HIV effort needs to be in line with targets set by PEPFAR. Furthermore, PEPFAR noted that they were critical to Kenya's delayed release of its 'population-based HIV impact assessment survey', which PEPFAR argued is needed to understand the state of Kenya's HIV epidemic. They noted also that a possible concern was the increasingly hostile environment emerging toward vulnerable populations in Tanzania as well as 'the country's program under-performance in some areas of its response' (Green, 2019). Leveraging progress toward the 90-90-90 targets as well as concerns over human rights and economic responsibility, PEPFAR has been able to reorient their efforts toward the 13 countries in its new strategy. This highlights the well-known problem of global health partnerships which are often analyzed as less partnership and more 'clientism' and 'global health diplomacy' wherein power is brokered through developmental and humanitarian aid (Adams, Novotny, & Leslie, 2008; Feldman & Ticktin, 2010; N. J. Kenworthy, 2014; N. J. Kenworthy & Parker, 2014). It also sheds light on the power of the 90-90-90 targets as metrics that serve to divide recipient countries into those who are, on the one hand, 'keeping the pace' and 'on track', and, on the other hand, those who are 'lagging behind' and 'not keeping the pace'. By utilizing progress toward epidemic control, PEPFAR can leverage power by threatening to or actually cutting funding to recipient countries.

A case in point is South Africa. South Africa is not a priority country, yet it has the largest HIV epidemic in the world and, as such, has received funds from PEPFAR. As an article in *Business Live* notes, South Africa had received about $670 million in fiscal year 2018. Yet PEPFAR noted in a letter that 'progress has been grossly sub-optimal and insufficient to reach epidemic control'; thus, PEPFAR would cut funding to $400 million for fiscal year 2019 (Green, 2019). The resulting tension can be seen in the outcry from activists in South Africa who noted that patients in South Africa should not fall victim to the dysfunctions of the South African health system and that the cuts might undermine the HIV efforts in the countries (Green, 2019).

PEPFAR was not the only one to adopt the new strategy of focusing on strategic interventions that would yield maximum impact. As Sara Davis notes, countries and organizations were told to cut unnecessary expenditures, use evidence-based interventions and show rapid progress toward the 90-90-90 targets (Davis, 2020). In an economic and political climate where programs are expected to 'do more with less', a renewed focus on targeting 'the right people and the right places' has emerged. In a book that chronicles what the end of AIDS narrative has come to signify, this is a significant point. Even though the case of PEPFAR is mainly concerned with high-prevalence countries in Sub-Saharan Africa, much of the same rationale of 'targeted HIV interventions' that are strategic and will maximize impact is found in the US, UK and Europe.

The focus on strategic interventions that would yield maximum impact has meant that the language of cost-effectiveness has come to dominate the end of AIDS narrative. The focus on the right places and the right people is, of course, part of this. With the implementation of the 90-90-90 targets, the end of AIDS could be scaled to fit any location and any population, i.e., subsets could be analyzed according to their progress along with the 90-90-90 targets as well as any geographical unit as long as the data was available. This has meant an increase in focus on data-gathering as well as establishing data infrastructures that can collect and monitor progress. In turn, using epidemiological data in combination with various emerging mapping technologies means that health care authorities could produce 'heat maps' or 'hot spots' to show where the epidemic is concentrated and then position clinics, hospitals and outreach programs where they are most needed (Davis, 2020). Space has emerged once again as an important focal point in HIV efforts. While space has always been part and parcel of the HIV epidemic, elegantly illustrated through the work of Lukas Engelmann (Engelmann, 2018), the novelty of the current focus on space lies in how indicators such as the 90-90-90 targets are being combined with epidemiological data, novel epidemiological mapping techniques such as GPS-assisted technologies and 'big data'.

However, in this new era of the coming of the end of AIDS, space is not the only topic that has received a new focus. Since the beginning of the HIV epidemic, sexual behavior has been a key focal point. Sexual behavior has been linked to certain population groups, and thus tracking and monitoring 'high-risk behavior' as well as prevalence and incidence rates within certain sub-sections of the population is part of HIV preventive efforts. Yet in the new end of AIDS narrative, as it has emerged through the language of the 90-90-90 targets, the focus on monitoring sub-populations and their progress along the 90-90-90 continuum is highlighted in several strategies. In a comment on the *Lancet-UNAIDS Commission*, Lo and Horton write that 'our Commission calls for all aspects of a comprehensive AIDS response to be funded and *targeted* where they will make the most difference, either in *geographical hotspots* or among *populations most at risk* of HIV' (Lo & Horton, 2015:107, my emphasis). The same has been echoed by UNAIDS which has called for programs to focus on 'location and population'. PEPFAR has also stated that there is a need to do 'the right things in the right places at the right time' and the Global Fund adds to this by saying there is a need to 'target resources to areas with the greatest need'.

The end of AIDS envisioned through the 90-90-90 targets thus opens up a very specific frame for talking about and implementing programs and interventions. These are often contingent upon data-driven epidemiology, cost-effectiveness models and the notion that interventions need to be targeted. To 'end AIDS' implies a collective form of action that is both global in reach and local in how it is implemented. Such a collective narrative of ending AIDS can fruitfully be analyzed as a form of *synchronization*, both in terms of synchronized actions but also as the synchronization of various spatio-temporal locales. The universal ambitions of the 90-90-90 targets, for instance, alludes to this global synchronized ambition of ending AIDS everywhere with the *same tools of synchronization* – that is, the path of the 90-90-90 targets.

With the introduction of the TasP paradigm which the 90-90-90 targets build on, a new way of tracking the end of AIDS has come about. By quantifying these goals, the global response to the HIV epidemic has become geared more toward counting and measuring progress through numbers that respond to the 90-90-90 targets. Indeed, as UNAIDS states: 'the old saying "What gets measured gets done" may be a cliché, but is still very true for the response to HIV'.[2] In turning to the 90-90-90 targets, a new norm within the global effort to 'bend the arc of the epidemic' was born. As the UNAIDS states,

> the 90–90–90 targets have become a central pillar of the global quest to end the AIDS epidemic. The targets reflect a fundamental shift in the world's approach to HIV treatment, moving it away from a focus on the number of people accessing antiretroviral therapy and toward the importance of maximizing viral suppression among people living with HIV.
>
> (UNAIDS, 2017a:8)

In the quote from the UNAIDS, the universal ambition and usefulness of the 90-90-90 targets are highlighted. Furthermore, the quote also highlights a new way of not only understanding how to best control, contain and even end the AIDS epidemic, but it also highlights that these targets are 'global' in their scope. This usage of the global and the world as space wherein the 90-90-90 targets are to be rolled out and used can be seen, I argue, as a universalizing norm of the 90-90-90 targets. Furthermore, this framing of the global utility of the 90-90-90 targets not only spatializes the implementation of these targets across the entire globe, but it also stipulates that the 90-90-90 targets become a global way of *counting* and *tracking* the *progress* of ending AIDS. Thus, a new spatio-temporal configuration of how to both *track and count* the progress toward ending AIDS is born.

The logic of track and count through the 90-90-90 targets points to the importance given to the universality of metrics in global health (Adams, 2016) and, specifically, in HIV/AIDS efforts. With the launch of the fast track strategy, UNAIDS underlined the importance of numerical targets by stating that 'targets drive progress', 'targets promote accountability', and finally, that targets underscore ending the AIDS epidemic is 'achievable' (UNAIDS, 2014a:11). The notion that numerical targets promote accountability is particularly striking here. Since funding is scarce for the global HIV effort, numerical targets also act as disciplinary metrics. Agencies such as the Global Fund, UNAIDS and local organizations that receive funds from, for instance, PEPFAR need to show progress along the 90-90-90 cascade to argue both for success as well as replenishments of their funds from donors. In so doing, we see the traces of what has been called 'audit culture' wherein data, targets and indicators have become key in monitoring success and disciplining failure (Shore, 2008; Shore & Wright, 1999, 2015).

Numerical targets such as the 90-90-90 targets also provide the global HIV effort with a tool that professes to be scalable and translatable across the globe. By this I mean that the 90-90-90 targets can be used at different scales (community, city, state, nation, region, global) and can be implemented anywhere regardless of geographical location, i.e. they work in any location. In this way, the 90-90-90 targets also offer a tool that makes the HIV epidemic commensurable across different scales and locations. Put differently, the 90-90-90 targets provide a set of targets that flattens the many differences that exist within the global HIV epidemic. We often talk about 'the HIV epidemic' in the singular, however, there are vast geographical differences, as well as socio-political and cultural differences that influence, drive and shape the HIV epidemic across the globe. Talking about the HIV epidemic in the singular allows for political focus, consolidates solidarity and points to some similarities across the globe. Yet it also risks flattening differences and homogenizes a very diverse epidemic that perhaps should be written in the plural. Either way, the 90-90-90 targets offer a way of making measurements commensurable across the globe in the efforts to end AIDS. These goals have provided a universal set of targets that are seemingly neutral and able to track progress toward the end of AIDS.

However, the perceived universality of numerical metrics such as the 90-90-90 targets is also important as a rhetorical device wherein the numbers can synchronize various actors in the global HIV/AIDS effort. Leclerc-Madlala et al. have, in the context of the introduction of the 90-90-90 targets within PEPFAR, commented that 'the task of getting a vastly heterogeneous global AIDS community on-board for the project of ending AIDS required consensus building, not only to establish support for the 2030 vision but also to establish a common language for the project' (Leclerc-Madlala et al., 2018:974). This common language, I argue, was the introduction of the 90-90-90 targets: numerical metrics that were perceived to be able to transcend the local epidemic variations and the heterogeneous cultural, economic and political contexts that the HIV epidemic is embedded within.

What Leclerc-Madlala et al. call a common language might also be read as a way of making the different manifestations of the HIV epidemic commensurable across the globe. Paraphrasing Dalsgaard, who has worked on the notion of commensurability concerning carbon, we can state that the 90-90-90 targets provide a set of universal metrics that seem to be able to 'transform different qualities within the HIV epidemic into a common set of metrics' (Dalsgaard, 2013). The differences within the global HIV epidemic are made commensurable through the 90-90-90 targets and allows for comparability across all scales. In this way, the 90-90-90 targets also act as a new standardized way of tracking the progress toward the end of AIDS. Standardization is, of course, a key aspect of making the world commensurable, and as Theodore Porter has noted, the process of standardization is often conducted through recourse to numerical metrics and statistics (Porter, 1986, 1996). There is, of course, a broad range of standardization techniques within the HIV epidemic ranging from the standardization of HIV tests, treatment guidelines, epidemiological categorization and other protocols and technologies. Yet, as Espeland and Stevens note, 'what distinguishes commensuration from other forms of standardization is the common metric it provides' (Espeland & Stevens, 1998:316). My argument is that the 90-90-90 targets provide the global HIV effort with precisely this form of commensuration through a common set of metrics. The common language becomes a way of making the many local HIV epidemics commensurable across space and differences, rendering these local differences comparable through a common set of metrics.

Sara Davis has noted this in a slightly different, yet important way. She states that the Fast Track strategy, launched by UNAIDS, was not just a strategy for ending AIDS, but it was equally a communication tool (Davis, 2020). Building on the work of Baumann, she notes that the 'end of AIDS' is a form of storytelling that is narrated through these various models, projections, strategies and reports to com-pel and persuade undecided people to care and to act (Davis, 2020). Finally, Davis links the storytelling of the end of AIDS to the 'noble lie' told in Plato's narrative about the Republic; here storytelling acts as an inspiring myth that could per-suade people to think about each other as brothers, despite the reality of inequality (Davis, 2020). Like Sara Davis, I agree that to conceptualize the end of AIDS as a 'noble lie' is not to say that it was or is an immoral or dishonest narrative. Rather, it is to highlight that while the end of AIDS narrative and its objectives are real, and that it is a story meant to inspire people to take action, it also is important to take note of how this narrative produced certain blind spots as well as new signi-fying practices. One consequence of the 'myth' of ending AIDS was the ability to *synchronize* efforts through the utilization of the 90-90-90 targets.

Synchronizing the end of AIDS

The first step in this process of creating a common language and thus a common synchronizing framework was the dissemination of various national and interna-tional documents such as white papers, reports, memos from meetings, scientific modeling, statistics, charts and, finally, high meeting declarations and concrete policy guidelines and strategies. Amongst this cascade of numbers and papers, we find reports such as the UNAIDS' *Fast Track: Ending the AIDS epidemic by 2030* (UNAIDS, 2014a); UNAIDS' *Ending AIDS: Progress toward the 90-90-90 targets* (UNAIDS, 2017a); UNAIDS' *Miles to go. Closing gaps, breaking barriers, righting injustices* (UNAIDS, 2018a); PEPFAR's *Blueprint* as well as PEPFAR's *PEPFAR 3.0* strategy. These are but a small sample of the documents that have gone into creating the common language that Leclerc-Madlala et al. point to. Moreover, at the heart of this common language for talking about the end of AIDS lies three numbers: 90-90-90. The function that these three figures have is deeply linked to two interrelated issues: the first, that the work of synchroniz-ing the global effort to end AIDS relies on an active acknowledgment that ART could bring about the end of AIDS if only scaled up; and the second, that countries need to commit themselves to specific targets and intervention and timelines to make this happen (Leclerc-Madlala et al., 2018:974). This last point is crucial, for it marks the temporal effect that these targets, in combination with deadlines for reaching these targets, have. In effect, the 90-90-90 targets become devices that not only counts specific subjects, i.e. people knowing their HIV status, people who are on ART and people who are virally suppressed, but they also become timekeeping devices that *count down toward the end of AIDS concerning the lin-ear progress toward either 2020 or 2030 depending on the frame of temporality they are embedded in.*

This common language of 90-90-90 targets relates to Jordheim and Wigen's argument for the creation of a synchronized international order. They state that

International order is also temporal order based on the alignment of more precisely, the synchronization of the multiple times at work on a global scale.

Synchronicity between cultures, languages, and policies does not emerge by itself. To create temporal orderings on a global scale requires work: political, social, and linguistic. Some work of synchronization is performed by technological innovations such as clocks, trains, satellites, etc. Another set of tools, however, is linguistic, made up of concepts used to create historical and political time understandable and workable.

(Jordheim & Wigen, 2018)

Transported to the case of the 90-90-90 targets and the end of AIDS, we might claim that the international order within the HIV effort is increasingly predicated upon the alignment of national progress toward the 90-90-90 targets. In the past, this was more aligned with epidemiological metrics, such as prevalence in the population, in general, and, to a certain degree, within key populations. Now we see a realignment along the 90-90-90 continuum. Furthermore, the 90-90-90 targets can be seen as a way of synchronizing various regional, national and local HIV temporalities with each other. They create a way of understanding the political temporal order within today's HIV history. Part of this synchronization is technical, such as viral mapping, epidemiological reporting, data collection, data networks, etc. Other parts are conceptual, such as the HIV crisis or HIV progress. They are, however, linked directly to the 90-90-90 targets which serve as a nexus for the synchronization of the end of AIDS.

The common language created by the 90-90-90 targets and the end of AIDS narrative is, as such, also a common synchronized conception of time and progress. While UNAIDS and PEPFAR, for instance, acknowledge the many local variations of the HIV epidemic as it is spread out across geographical space, the 90-90-90 targets seems to introduce a universal way of counting, tracking and checking the progress of the epidemic regardless of local variations; in short, it is a universal language to understand and synchronize efforts in ending AIDS.

This is important, as it has allowed not only for the tracking of the progress toward ending AIDS, but it also has allowed for a universal frame of reference which allows for comparison *between* various nations as well as *within* them through both *diachronic and synchronic* dimensions. UNAIDS alludes to as much through quotes such as

The latest epidemiological estimates and program data from 168 countries in all regions reveal progress and gaps across the HIV testing and treatment cascade. Changes in HIV policy since 2014 were also reported by countries, as were the development and roll-out of innovations in technology and service delivery.

(UNAIDS, 2017a:9)

The 90-90-90 targets thus represent a *synchronization through counting* on a global scale. However, this synchronization is not only a synchronization of actions taken to end AIDS such as the scale-up of testing, treating and ensuring that PLHIV reach undetectable viral loads; rather this synchronization of actions is also *timebound* as the UNAIDS states: 'As the world approaches the midway point between the 2014 launch of the 90–90–90 targets and their December 2020 deadline, UNAIDS has reviewed the progress made' (UNAIDS, 2017a:9). Time is thus essential. As such, local communities and nations must synchronize their efforts both through the implementation and scale-up of public health initiatives which are in line with the 90-90-90 targets as well as synchronizing their horizon for ending AIDS with that of the UNAIDS 90-90-90 deadline and, ultimately, the UN *Sustainable Development Goals* deadline of 2030. This deadline is also invoked by the progress report on the 90-90-90 targets:

> Consistent with the commitment to leave no one behind in transforming our world: the 2030 agenda for sustainable development, UNAIDS, and its partners reviewed and synthesized country data and studies that revealed the particular challenges and strategies for securing the full preventive and therapeutic benefits of antiretroviral therapy.
>
> (UNAIDS, 2017a: 9)

Action and time are synchronized; space and temporality are subsumed under this new universal way of tracking and counting (down toward) the end of AIDS, and the global is evoked as the space in which this universal timeline of progress is now unfolding.

Formulated through theories of temporality and the philosophy of history, we might state that the 90-90-90 targets allow for a universal time-space that is linear and homogenous, wherein progress is to be tracked exclusively through universal metrics represented by the 90-90-90 targets. Through the universal and global 90-90-90 targets and their subsequent activities, a universal narrative of progress toward a goal, a deadline nonetheless, is formulated. Through this universal time-space, different localities, different spaces and, we might add here, different temporalities are synchronized through initiatives such as the many self-reporting mechanisms wherein nations are encouraged to report their progress toward ending AIDS. Other initiatives include the 'Fast Track Cities' which is 'a global partnership between cities and municipalities around the world and four core partners – the International Association of Providers of AIDS Care (IAPAC), the Joint United Nations Programme on HIV/AIDS (UNAIDS), the United Nations Human Settlements Programme (UN-Habitat), and the City of Paris'.[3] The Fast Track Cities initiative now includes 'more than 250 cities and municipalities that are committed to attaining the UNAIDS 90-90-90 targets by 2020' and through 'the principle of data transparency, the initiative includes a Fast-Track Cities Global Web Portal that allows cities to report on their progress against the fast-track and other targets'.[4] This clearly shows the synchronization of the efforts made across the globe to reach the 90-90-90 targets within 2020 as well as a way to compare progress and note who is lagging behind (not keeping the pace *en route* to ending AIDS). These initiatives, global in scope and stretching from Nairobi in Kenya to Miami in the US and from Santiago in Chile to Bangkok in Thailand, allow for the 'synchronicity of the non-synchronous' (Jordheim, 2017:66). My strong argument here is that the 90-90-90 targets should not only be seen as a way of counting the progress toward the end of AIDS or as a synchronizing effort in establishing a universal standard of HIV treatment and prevention. Rather, I argue that we can see this as also the emergence of a new universal and standardized *temporality* within the periodization of the HIV epidemic. A temporality or time structure which insists on the synchronization of both lived lives and various practices, but also the synchronization of the *many times* embedded within the HIV epidemic and in the millions of people who live with HIV and even the many millions who are considered to be at risk of HIV.

Reviewing the numbers: what about the 10-10-10?

The 90-90-90 targets seem ambitious and bold both in what the numbers say and what the model stipulates. Yet the 90-90-90 targets are also filled with embedded shortcomings. The targets themselves indeed anticipate that within a step of the targets there will be those who do not get tested, those who do not access treatment and, finally, those who will not achieve viral load suppression. In addition to this, the numbers of people who will not reach the targets grow from one metric to the next. If we use the denominator of *all people living with HIV*, then the 90-90-90 targets' anticipated shortcomings translates to 90-81-73; thus, the targets themselves acknowledge implicitly that 10% won't get tested, 19% will not receive treatment and 27% will not be virally suppressed.

Vincanne Adams et al. has pointed to the function of anticipation in global health care and technoscience (Adams, Murphy, & Clarke, 2009), and the 90-90-90 targets seem to be an example of such a politics of anticipation. On the one hand, UNAIDS envisions that the path to an end to the HIV epidemic is through the 90-90-90 targets; however, at the same time, the very mathematical model of reaching the 90-90-90 targets anticipates and produces its outside. In terms of synchronicity, it produces its non-synchronous outside – the people who are anticipated to be left 'outside' of the fulfillment of the 90-90-90 targets.

This begs the question, states Judith Auerbach: 'who are the other 10-10-10, or rather, who are the other 10-19-27 who are not reached or engaged in the treatment cascade?' (Auerbach, 2019:100). Who are the ones left behind within the model and who is not synchronized through the apparatus of the 90-90-90 targets?

It is outside the scope of this chapter to answer this question, but a summary is to provide a critique of the 90-90-90 targets both as the alleged guarantee toward the end of AIDS as well as noting the shortcomings of the model.

In brief, Auerbach points out that there are vast differences globally in terms of people knowing their status, but that in 2017, data showed that out of 82 countries (representing 92% of the global HIV burden), only 4 had reached the first target, and only 18 had reached 70%–89% of people knowing their HIV status (Auerbach, 2019:100). Similarly, global numbers from 2017 showed that for the second target, accessing treatment, there were large gaps and differences across the globe. Treatment numbers ranged from 85% in Western Europe and North America to 29% in the Middle East and North Africa (Auerbach, 2019:101).

However, broken down on regional levels, there are disparities even within countries with a generally high level of access to ARVs, as I will show later.

Finally, the story is not much different for the last target, people who are virally suppressed. Here too we find large global differences in how many achieve viral suppression. In the Middle East, for instance, only 22% of PLHIV were reported as having a suppressed viral load, while, in North America and Western Europe the numbers were as high as 65% (UNAIDS, 2018). Once again, the local differences here are stark as well. While North America has seen increasing numbers of people reaching viral suppression, disparities still exist; data from San Francisco, for instance, show that young people and women (both cis and transgender) are less likely to achieve viral suppression than older adults and men (Garcia, Aragon, & Scheer, 2017). Finally, another problem with the 90-90-90 targets lies in the linear understanding or portrayal of reaching these goals. On the national level, this can mean that countries fall in and out of the list of countries that have reached these numbers as numbers can fluctuate and are time-bound. For people, this can mean that they are in and out of care, and this influences how viral suppression is maintained (Auerbach, 2019:101). HIV treatment and care is not a linear process – either at the national level or the personal level of people living with HIV. The end of AIDS, barring an effective vaccine or cure, is thus not an *event* but a continual process that needs to be understood as such.

This also leads to a final critique of the 90-90-90 targets: namely that the 90-90-90 targets firmly focuses on treatment. While treatment is key and crucial to the overall success of the HIV efforts, several scholars, community activists and affected community members have drawn attention to the need for *other* indicators and targets that go beyond the treatment paradigm. Some have drawn attention to the need for a 'fourth 90' which is often conceptualized through the framework of quality of life (Harris, Rabkin, & El-Sadr, 2018; Lazarus et al., 2016). As Auerback suggests, good health and quality of life are not part of the 90-90-90 targets and data on this amongst people living with HIV are not collected as part of the official UNAIDS framework, thus it is not measured (Auerbach, 2019:101). Since viral load suppression for most people living with HIV is not the end-all be-all, it is important to consider that it is possible for people living with HIV that 'quality of life' might involve discontinuation of ARV, if they tire of it or if it is a reminder of chronic living where adherence is expected to continue throughout their lives (Auerbach, 2019:101). This critique reveals the many tensions that have come to occupy HIV-related global health efforts and how metrics and indicators have come to take center stage on the road toward the end of AIDS. It also should remind us that these aspects of the HIV epidemic are not only political or even technical in nature. They are highly lived and social phenomena. Finally, the usage of and reliance on the 90-90-90 targets also highlight how the world of HIV is made commensurable through metrics that, at times, obfuscate as much as they illuminate.

As such, the establishment of a universal and standardized way of counting and tracking the progress toward the end of AIDS has been fundamental in the synchronization of efforts to end AIDS across the globe. It has also been, as I have argued, fundamental in the formation of a new temporality which introduces a universal, homogenous and linear temporality marked by two clearly defined end-points – 2020 and 2030 – which the global HIV prevention efforts must synchronize themselves against. This allows for comparison as we have stated, through synchronic and diachronic frames of references both within nations, even cities, but also across them. Several cities engaged in the Fast-Track Cities Initiative have also reached, or are close to reaching, the 90–90–90 targets, including Amsterdam, Melbourne, New York City and Paris (UNAIDS, 2017b:10). This comparative framework thus allows for tracking progress but also masking the many fine-grained disparities which exist within these localized spaces. Case in point is New York City, wherein the city itself might be close to achieving the 90-90-90 targets but disparities that cut across ethnic and racial lines still exist. As the Henry Kaiser Family Foundation (KFF) states: 'While many Blacks (84%) are diagnosed, 46% remain in regular care, and fewer (43%) are virally suppressed. Blacks also may be less likely to sustain viral suppression and may experience longer periods with higher viral loads, compared to other groups' (KFF, 2020). This is presented in detail in the New York City Department of Health and Mental Hygiene report for 2017. While 80 percent of all PLHIV in NYC were virally suppressed, only 75 percent of all transgender women were suppressed and 76 percent of women were suppressed (NYDOH, 2019). When broken down by racial categories, the figures read that 76 percent of Blacks were virally suppressed; 81 percent of Hispanics were virally suppressed; 90 percent of the White PLHIV had achieved viral suppression; 87 percent of Asian/Pacific Islanders had achieved this and finally, 70 percent of Native Americans had achieved the goal of becoming virally suppressed. If we look at the UK and London, we can also discern how the race toward the 90-90-90 targets and its global synchronizing efforts are celebrated but hide disparities. London was heralded as 'the first global city to exceed UNAIDS 95-95-95 ambitions' (Healthy London Partnership, 2018) in 2018. London achieved the targets of 95-98-97 respectively along the 90-90-90 continuum. This was lauded by Dr. Tom Coffey, Mayoral Health Advisor in London as 'London is leading the way when it comes to tackling HIV' and that London was committed to 'ending new infections by 2030' (Healthy London Partnership, 2018). While the progress that London has made along with the 90-90-90 targets, one striking disparity can be teased out by the Public Health England (PHE) 2017 report. Here we can read that while London and England, in general, have managed to exceed the UNAIDS targets, late diagnosis is still a concern for PLHIV and, in particular, amongst 'Black African heterosexual' men and women of whom 52 percent and 69 percent, respectively, were diagnosed late (PHE, 2018). Since a late diagnosis of HIV is associated with higher mortality and morbidity rates as well as 'have been at risk of passing on HIV to partners if having sex without condoms' (PHE, 2018), late diagnosis is a particularly worrisome aspect of HIV surveillance. The point here is not to take away from the important work that London and England have done through its HIV treatment and prevention work; rather, it is to highlight that a target-based system with a temporal horizon, albeit important, still glosses over important disparities within local epidemics.

Another key critique of the 'politics of counting' comes from the work of Sara Davis' notion of 'the politics of the *uncounted*' (Davis, 2017, 2020; Davis, Goedel, Emerson, & Guven, 2017). Davis' work points to how the governing HIV efforts through the usage of metrics as guides can obfuscate as much as they purport to illuminate. Case in point from Davis' work is how so-called 'key population estimates' are used in establishing a baseline metric for counting 'key population size' within countries. In brief, the calculation of key populations is based on statistical calculations based on national and international surveys as well as demographic data. Through calculation, nations provide an estimate of the 'prevalence' of how many men who have sex with men or transgender women there are within a given population; based on this baseline, one can calculate how many percent of men who have sex with men have tested positive for HIV. However, as Davis' work shows, many nations, in particular nations that have punitive laws against sex between men, underreport the size of the population that would be categorized as men who have sex with men (Davis, 2017; Davis et al., 2017). This problem is even more visible in categorizing transgender women for instance. Thus, the politics of counting as envisioned by the 90-90-90 targets should be interrogated just as much by the politics of the *uncounted*. Rendered invisible in the data also means that entire communities are being left behind and outside of the synchronized efforts to end AIDS. The metrics themselves produce communities of people who then become *outside of synchronization*.

Problematizing the role of indicators and metrics such as the 90-90-90 targets also involves an apparent anticipated result of the 90-90-90 targets. While the 90-90-90 targets were never intended to 'end AIDS' per se, only to achieve 'epidemic control', they still provide an important vista into how these targets also produce their outside, their non-synchronous subjects.

My main concern though is to highlight how the establishment of the 90-90-90 targets and its subsequent counting can be seen as one of the tools or practices of synchronizing the end of AIDS narrative.

The work of synchronization that the 90-90-90 targets do also includes the introduction of a framework for comparison. That is, since the 90-90-90 targets bring with them a universal language and a universal horizon of time, it allows for comparison between and across various geographical units. These units of comparison are continental, regional, national and even local and city level (UNAIDS, 2017a; UNAIDS, 2018a, 2019). In light of this comparative optic, temporality is also introduced through temporal linguistic markers such as 'lagging', 'keeping the pace' and 'being off track', but also through charts and diagrams which introduces diagrammatic thinking around progress and the nature of tracking the end of AIDS.

I have in this chapter provided an abridged history toward the end of AIDS as it has emerged in the wake of the 90-90-90 targets. In doing so I have also teased out how the 90-90-90 targets came to be and how these targets, numerical as they are, also provide a narrative, a common language for diverse actors to rally around. One of the key points has been to highlight how, in the wake of an indicator-driven, data-dependent end to AIDS, as well as fiscal austerity, there has emerged a renewed focus on specific people and specific places. The remainder of the book focuses on how targeted efforts, be they mapping technology or targeted prevention campaigns, produce various signifying practices. As such, it is to the new technologies of geospatial mapping and epidemiological surveillance that the next chapter will be dedicated.

Notes

1 See the AVERT HIV timeline; https://www.avert.org/professionals/history-hiv-aids/overview
2 See the UNAIDS' webpage; http://www.unaids.org/en/topic/data
3 See the Fast Track Cities webpage; http://www.iapac.org/fast-track-cities/about-fast-track/
4 See the Fast Track Cities webpage; http://www.iapac.org/fast-track-cities/about-fast-track/

References

Adams, V. (2016). *Metrics: What counts in global health.* Durham, NC: Duke University Press.

Adams, V., Murphy, M., & Clarke, A. E. (2009). Anticipation: Technoscience, life, affect, temporality. *Subjectivity, 28*(1), 246–265.

Adams, V., Novotny, T. E., & Leslie, H. (2008). Global health diplomacy. *Medical Anthropology, 27*(4), 315–323.

Angotti, N. (2012). Testing differences: The implementation of Western HIV testing norms in sub-Saharan Africa. *Culture, Health and Sexuality, 14*(4), 365–378.

Auerbach, J. D. (2019). Getting to zero begins with getting to ten. *Journal of Acquired Immune Deficiency Syndromes (1999), 82*(2), S99.

Battacharya, S. (2003). Worst ever year for HIV, says expert. *The New Scientist, 2003.*

Beer, D. (2016). *Metric power.* Berlin: Springer.

Center for Disease Control. (1999). MMWR, *Supplement, December 31, 1999 / 48(SU01);23-7.*

Cohen, J. (2011a). HALTING HIV/AIDS epidemics. *Science, 334*(6061), 1338–1340. doi:10.1126/science.334.6061.1338.

Cohen, J. (2011b). *HIV treatment as prevention.* American Association for the Advancement of Science.

Cohen, M. S., Chen, Y. Q., McCauley, M., Gamble, T., Hosseinipour, M. C., Kumarasamy, N. ... Pilotto, J. H. (2011). Prevention of HIV-1 infection with early antiretroviral therapy. *New England Journal of Medicine, 365*(6), 493–505.

Cohen, M. S., McCauley, M., & Gamble, T. R. (2012). HIV treatment as prevention and HPTN 052. *Current Opinion in HIV and AIDS, 7*(2), 99.

Dalsgaard, S. (2013). The commensurability of carbon: Making value and money of climate change. *HAU: Journal of Ethnographic Theory, 3*(1), 80–98.

Davis, S. L. (2017). The uncounted: Politics of data and visibility in global health. *The International Journal of Human Rights, 21*(8), 1144–1163.

Davis, S. L. (2020). *The uncounted: Politics of data in global health.* Cambridge: Cambridge University Press.

Davis, S. L., Goedel, W. C., Emerson, J., & Guven, B. S. (2017). Punitive laws, key population size estimates, and Global AIDS Response Progress Reports an ecological study of 154 countries. *Journal of the International AIDS Society, 20*(1), 21386.

Engebretsen, E., Heggen, K., Das, S., Farmer, P., & Ottersen, O. P. (2016). Paradoxes of sustainability with consequences for health. *Lancet Global Health, 4*(4), e225–e226.

Engebretsen, E., Heggen, K., & Ottersen, O. P. (2017). The Sustainable Development Goals: Ambiguities of accountability. *Lancet, 389*(10067), 365.

Engelmann, L. (2018). *Mapping AIDS: Visual histories of an enduring epidemic.* Cambridge: Cambridge University Press.

Epstein, S. (1996). *Impure Science: AIDS, activism, and the politics of knowledge* (Vol. 7). Berkeley, CA: University of California Press.

Espeland, W. N., & Stevens, M. L. (1998). Commensuration as a social process. *Annual Review of Sociology, 24*(1), 313–343.

Farmer, P. (2004). An anthropology of structural violence. *Current Anthropology, 45*(3), 305–325. doi:10.1086/382250.

Farmer, P. (2006). *AIDS and accusation: Haiti and the geography of blame.* Berkeley, CA: University of California Press.

Feldman, I., & Ticktin, M. (2010). *In the name of humanity: The government of threat and care.* Durham, NC: Duke University Press.

Garcia, B., Aragon, T., & Scheer, S. (2017). HIV epidemiology annual report 2016. San Francisco Department of Public Health Population Health Division.

Granich, R. M., Gilks, C. F., Dye, C., De Cock, K. M., & Williams, B. G. (2009). Universal voluntary HIV testing with immediate antiretroviral therapy as a strategy for elimination of HIV transmission: A mathematical model. *Lancet, 373*(9657), 48–57.

Granich, R., Williams, B., Montaner, J., & Zuniga, J. M. (2017). 90-90-90 and ending AIDS: Necessary and feasible. *Lancet, 390*(10092), 341–343.

Green, A. (2019). What's behind PEPFAR's funding cut threats? *Devex.* Retrieved from https://www.devex.com/news/what-s-behind-pepfar-s-funding-cut-threats-95053.

Hafner, T., & Shiffman, J. (2012). The emergence of global attention to health systems strengthening. *Health Policy and Planning, 28*(1), 41–50.

Harris, T. G., Rabkin, M., & El-Sadr, W. M. (2018). Achieving the fourth 90: healthy aging for people living with HIV. *AIDS (London, England), 32*(12), 1563.

Healthy London Partnership (2018). London the first global city to exceed UNAIDS 95-95-95 ambitions. Retrieved from https://www.healthylondon.org/london-first-global-city-to-exceed-unaids-ambitions/.

Jordheim, H. (2017). Synchronizing the world: Synchronism as historiographical practice, then and now. *History of the Present, 7*(1), 59–95.

Jordheim, H., & Wigen, E. (2018). Conceptual synchronisation: From progress to crisis. *Millennium, 46*(3), 421–439.

Kasier Family Foundation. (2020). Black Americans and HIV/AIDS: The basics. Retrieved from https://www.kff.org/hivaids/fact-sheet/black-americans-and-hivaids-the-basics/

Kenworthy, N. J. (2014). Global health: The debts of gratitude. *Women's Studies Quarterly, 42*(1/2), 69–85.

Kenworthy, N. J., & Parker, R. (2014). *HIV scale-up and the politics of global health.* London, New York.

Kenworthy, N., Thomann, M., & Parker, R. (2018a). Critical perspectives on the 'end of AIDS'. *Global Public Health, 13*(8), 1–3.

Kenworthy, N., Thomann, M., & Parker, R. (2018b). From a global crisis to the 'end of AIDS': New epidemics of signification. *Global Public Health, 13*(8), 960–971.

Lachenal, G. (2013). "A genealogy of treatment as prevention (TASP): Prevention, therapy, and the tensions of public health in African history". In: *Global Health in Africa: Historical Perspectives on Disease Control (Perspectives on Global Health)* 1st Edition, edited by Tamara Vernic and James Webb, 70–91. Athens: Ohio University Press.

Lazarus, J. V., Safreed-Harmon, K., Barton, S. E., Costagliola, D., Dedes, N., del Amo Valero, J. … Porter, K. (2016). Beyond viral suppression of HIV–the new quality of life frontier. *BMC Medicine, 14*(1), 94.

Leclerc-Madlala, S., Broomhall, L., & Fieno, J. (2018). The 'end of AIDS'project: Mobilising evidence, bureaucracy, and big data for a final biomedical triumph over AIDS. *Global Public Health, 13*(8), 972–981.

Lo, S., & Horton, R. (2015). AIDS and global health: The path to sustainable development. *Lancet, 386*(9989), 106–108. doi:10.1016/S0140-6736(15)61040-6.

Luginaah, I. N., Yiridoe, E. K., & Taabazuing, M.-M. (2005). From mandatory to voluntary testing: Balancing human rights, religious and cultural values, and HIV/AIDS prevention in Ghana. *Social Science and Medicine, 61*(8), 1689–1700.

MacPhail, C. L., Pettifor, A., Coates, T., & Rees, H. (2008). "You must do the test to know your status": Attitudes to HIV voluntary counseling and testing for adolescents among South African youth and parents. *Health Education and Behavior, 35*(1), 87–104.

Michael, M., & Rosengarten, M. (2013). *Innovation and biomedicine: Ethics, evidence, and expectation in HIV*. Berlin: Springer.

Nattrass, N. (2014). Millennium development goal 6: AIDS and the international health agenda. *Journal of Human Development and Capabilities, 15*(2–3), 232–246.

Nattrass, N., & Gonsalves, G. (2009). Economics and the backlash against AIDS-specific funding.

Nattrass, N., & Gonsalves, G. (2010). AIDS funds: Undervalued. *Science, 330*(6001), 174–175.

New York City Deapartment of Public Health. (2019). Care and clinical status of people newly diagnosed with HIV and people living with HIV in New York City, 2018. Retrieved from https://www1.nyc.gov/assets/doh/downloads/pdf/dires/hiv-related-m edical-care.pdf.

Nguyen, V.-K., O'malley, J., & Pirkle, C. M. (2011). Remedicalizing an epidemic: From HIV treatment as prevention to HIV treatment is prevention. *AIDS, 25*(11), 1435.

PEPFAR. (2016). *Building a sustainable future*. PEPFAR, Washington, DC.

PEPFAR. (2017). *Strategy for accelerating HIV/AIDS epidemic control*. PEPFAR, Washington, DC.

PEPFAR. (2018). *PEPFAR 3.0. Controlling the epidemic: Delivering on the promise of an HIV free generation*. PEPFAR, Washington, DC.

Piot, P. (2003). *AIDS: The need for exceptional response to an unprecedented crisis*. Presidential Fellow Lecture. Washington, DC.

Porter, T. M. (1986). *The rise of statistical thinking, 1820–1900*. Princeton, NJ: Princeton University Press.

Porter, T. M. (1996). *Trust in numbers: The pursuit of objectivity in science and public life*. Princeton, NJ: Princeton University Press.

Public Health England. (2018). Progress toward ending the HIV epidemic in the United Kingdom. Retrieved from https://assets.publishing.service.gov.uk/government/upl oads/system/uploads/attachment_data/file/821273/Progress_toward_ending_the_HIV _epidemic_in_the_UK.pdf.

Rodger, A. J., Cambiano, V., Bruun, T., Vernazza, P., Collins, S., Van Lunzen, J. ... Beloukas, A. (2016). Sexual activity without condoms and the risk of HIV transmission in serodifferent couples when the HIV-positive partner is using suppressive antiretroviral therapy. *JAMA, 316*(2), 171–181.

Rosengarten, M., & Michael, M. (2009). The performative function of expectations in translating treatment to prevention: The case of HIV pre-exposure prophylaxis, or PrEP. *Social Science and Medicine, 69*(7), 1049–1055.

Sangaramoorthy, T. (2018). Chronicity, crisis, and the 'end of AIDS'. *Global Public Health, 13*(8), 982–996.

Shore, C. (2008). Audit culture and illiberal governance: Universities and the politics of accountability. *Anthropological Theory, 8*(3), 278–298.

Shore, C., & Wright, S. (1999). Audit culture and anthropology: Neo-liberalism in British higher education. *Journal of the Royal Anthropological Institute, 5*(4), 557–575.

Shore, C., & Wright, S. (2015). Governing by numbers: Audit culture, rankings and the new world order. *Social Anthropology, 23*(1), 22–28.

Sibanda, A. (2000). A nation in pain: Why the HIV/AIDS epidemic is out of control in Zimbabwe. *International Journal of Health Services, 30*(4), 717–738.

Sidibe, M. (2014). 90-90-90: A transformative agenda to leave no one behind. Retrieved from https://www.unaids.org/en/speeches/2014/20141025_SP_EXD_Vietnam_launch _of_909090_en.pdf.

Sidibé, M., Loures, L., & Samb, B. (2016). The UNAIDS. 90–90–90 target: A clear choice for ending AIDS and for sustainable health and development. *Journal of the International AIDS Society, 19*(1), 21133.

UNAIDS. (2000). UN Security Council Resolution 1308 (2000) on the Responsibility of the Security Council in the Maintenance of International Peace and Security. HIV/ AIDS and international peace-keeping operations, 1308.

UNAIDS. (2014). Fast-track: Ending the AIDS epidemic by 2030. UNAIDS/*JC2686*.

UNAIDS. (2017a). Ending AIDS: Progress toward the 90–90–90 targets.

UNAIDS. (2017b). Ending AIDS: Progress toward the 90-90-90 targets. *Global AIDS Update*.

UNAIDS. (2018). Miles to go—Closing gaps, breaking barriers, righting injustices, 268.

UNAIDS. (2019). Global AIDS Monitoring 2019. Indicators for the monitoring of the 2016 Political Declaration on Ending AIDS, 208.

WHO. (2006). *Bulletin of the World Health Organization*, Vol. 84, number 2, February, 81–160

Part II

'Hotspots', space, risk and surveillance

3 Viral load maps

The entanglements between the individual, the community and space

Introduction

If metrics and indicators have provided a powerful way of conceptualizing the end of AIDS, then maps have served as another modality in which to visualize both the history of the HIV epidemic and its epidemiological distribution across the globe. With the 90-90-90 target of achieving viral suppression amongst PLHIV, visualizing the progress toward the end of AIDS through maps has once again become a particularly influential way of 'knowing the epidemic'. The proliferation of various types of maps that report on the current HIV epidemic has become an increasingly popular way of tracking the progress toward the end of AIDS.

This and the next chapter interrogate the ways in which HIV science has increasingly taken space and place as its focal point in the name of ending AIDS. More specifically, I argue that space has become important as part of the emerging discourse of ending AIDS. Subsequently, space and place has emerged as both a problem area of the HIV epidemic and a potential space wherein surveillance and interventions can be implemented.

Epidemiological mapping of the HIV epidemic is far from a new field of study. Lukas Engelmann has delivered an exemplary study of the visual histories of the HIV/AIDS epidemic and the use of photography, maps and images of the HIV virus itself (Engelmann, 2018). Others, such as Adrian Guta and Marilou Gagnon, have looked at the intersections between viral suppression, mapping and technologies of medical surveillance as it has started to emerge in HIV public health initiatives (Gagnon & Guta, 2012a, 2012b, 2014). This chapter will follow some of the work that these scholars have done, but I will argue that the mapping of the HIV epidemic, as it is conducted today, is part and parcel not only of a visualization of the epidemic, but also a way of tracking progress toward the end of AIDS. This is important when we look at the many ways in which notions of surveillance and control as well as notions of responsibility and accountability are invoked. The mapping of the end of AIDS, I argue, entails the spatialization of a normative power which distributes responsibility, interventions and blame across geographical space according to metrics, such as viral load measurements or phylogenetic clusters of new HIV infections.

Epidemiological maps: spatializing disease and visualizing cases

Mapping diseases has a long history in public health initiatives and the governing of global, public and community health. One of the best-known examples of this is John Snow's famous mapping of the 1854 cholera epidemic in London. Snow, in his book *On the Mode of Communication of Cholera* (Snow, 1855), showed through case mappings of cholera cases in London how the disease spread and provided a 'diagram of the topography of the outbreak' as he said (Snow, 1855:45). By providing a map over London's 1854 cholera outbreak, Snow plotted deaths by cholera, affixing them to addresses on the map where they occurred, thus revealing a pattern of distribution of the outbreak. Snow's work was conducted by weaving together multiple sources of data, such as statistical data from tables, case histories and observations made about social behavior in several of London's districts. Maps such as John Snow's paved the way for a new way of framing and 'seeing spaces of disease'. Disease maps, as Engelmann calls them, 'allow for an indefinite number of assumptions, datasets, theories and critical inquiries to be applied to the spatio-temporal structure of an outbreak of a disease' (Engelmann, 2018:120). Stated differently, maps started to provide new and convincing ways of framing disease etiologies, patterns of distributions and their temporal speeds. Maps, when placed in seriality, offered a powerful way of not only visualizing disease distribution but also speed – that is, temporality. Epidemiological maps are scalar in nature, that is, they operate on different scales such as local, national, regional and global (Campbell, Cornish, & Skovdal, 2012). This is due to the nature of the epidemiological denominators, such as prevalence, incidence rates, mortality rates and morbidity rates, all deemed to be 'translatable' across any of these scales. Second of all, epidemiological maps allow for the placement of a disease on the ground in a two-dimensional space wherein these maps answer what Koch sees as three essential questions: 'where did this disease come from? How is it distributed? What is it?' (Koch, 2011; Koch & Koch, 2005). Epidemiological maps, Koch states, can be seen as devices which mediate a particular enactment of the disease in question; it is an assemblage of various forms of data sources which, while professing to tell a neutral story of the disease, nevertheless enact a particular ontological version of the disease (Koch, 2011).

> Through a map, particular qualities of space are interrogated as a means of understanding why an epidemic appeared in that specific mapped place. The map seems to ask its readers what allowed the epidemic to thrive in this place, and what can be learned from these particularities to contain further distribution.
>
> (Engelmann, 2018:107)

This has certainly been the case with the mapping of the HIV/AIDS epidemic as shown by both Engelmann (2018) and Pépin in his book *The Origins of AIDS* (Pépin, 2011; Pépin, 2013). Infectious diseases in particular have been the subject of various forms of disease mapping and have been a favored way of enacting the many global and national epidemics in both public health reports and in the media at large. Nancy Krieger states that 'despite epidemiology's longstanding concern with 'time, place and person', [...] 'place' had receded into the background by the mid-20th century, conceptually unmoored from increasingly influential etiologic frameworks based on characteristics of the individual' (Krieger, 2003:384). Yet with the emergence of new geographic information system (GIS) maps and big-data data analysis, epidemiology has once again turned to mapping as a way of offering a spatial analysis of various public health issues. This has not only allowed for the re-enchantment of the power of the disease map in terms of its ability to analyze spatial distributions and variation of disease and illness, but has also enabled epidemiologists to simulate, through geo-informatics, various epidemics and model epidemic spread, patterns and impacts (Lorway & Khan, 2014:53). HIV science has been quick to utilize these sorts of technologies both as tools of modelling epidemic spread and patterns and as a way of providing 'near real time' surveillance (Poon et al., 2016) of the spread and clustering of HIV.

Spatializing the end of AIDS: the role of the community viral load

By now the value of the viral load metric and its usage in clinical as well as public health initiative is understood. This metric is seen as the successful end point of HIV treatment for PLHIV. It is the continual process of adhering to ARVs on a daily basis and regular viral load testing at clinics. The viral load metric has become increasingly important both as a metric of individual health (low viral load metrics often indicate healthier immune system at the individual level); as an indicator of not being able to pass on HIV (a 'non-detectable' measurement at the individual level reduces the risk of sexually transmitting HIV to 'effectively no risk' as per the US CDC[1]); and finally, as a metric for evaluating community health and infectiousness in terms of what has been called 'community viral load' (Das et al., 2010; Herbeck & Tanser, 2016). As such, the viral load metric has a unique biopolitical function in that it entangles notions of being and staying healthy for the individual with the potential of the individual to pass on HIV, and finally, the infectiousness of entire communities. It thus exists on two levels in the biopolitical matrix of HIV governance: on the one hand, it targets individuals to adhere to ARVs thus, *individualizing* HIV governmentality; on the other hand, it 'massefies' the individual by acting as a metric for the total viral load of entire communities, thus acting upon populations as well as individuals.

Before getting ahead of ourselves, let us take a closer look at how community viral load (CVL) came to be such an important vector and, in particular, how it became the subject of epidemiological mapping.

Das et al. stated, in a study from 2010, that "community viral load was an aggregate biological measure of viral load for a particular geographic location – for example the city of San Francisco or a particular neighborhood – and for a particular group of people who share socio-demographic characteristics" (Das et al., 2010:2). In order to calculate community viral load within any specific group or area, there are two different measurements that one must take into account: one is the mean community viral load and the other is total community viral load (Das et al., 2010:2). Mean community viral load is defined as 'the average of the most recent VL of all reported HIV-positive individuals in a particular population' (Das et al., 2010:2). Total community viral load on the other hand is defined as 'the sum of the most recent VL of all reported HIV-positive individuals in a particular population' (Das et al., 2010:2). These two metrics allows for the determination of the mean average viral burden within a population or geographical area and the absolute level of the virus within a population or geographical area. After Das et al.'s study, several studies ensued and the notion that decreases in community viral load would lead to reduction in new HIV infections started to be seen as a valuable marker for the 'direct relationship between HIV concentration (in specific populations and geographical areas) and overall HIV incidence' (Gagnon & Guta, 2012b:473). As such, one of the outcomes of the concept of community viral load as predicator for reduction or increase in new HIV infections has been the scale-up of both HIV testing, viral load surveillance and the aforementioned reconceptualization of antiretroviral treatment as not only a treatment modality but also a preventive technology (Gagnon & Guta, 2012b:473). It should be mentioned that community viral load as an indicator for the decrease in new HIV infections amongst a particular population or geographical area has not been met without its share of criticism. Mostly, the critique has been about which mathematical formulation to use in determining the effect of community viral load levels as an indicator of HIV reduction (Tanser et al., 2017) and the 'disconnect' between population-based and individual-based HIV prevention (Baral et al., 2019). From a social science perspective, the criticism has focused on how community viral load measurements and their subsequent visualization and spatialization has engendered a politics of 'stigma and exclusion' (Gagnon & Guta, 2012a, 2012b, 2014).

The first studies of the usefulness of community viral loads in North America were conducted in the following cities: one in Vancouver (Montaner et al., 2010); another in San Francisco (Das et al., 2010); three in New York (Forgione & Torzian, 2012; Laraque et al., 2013; Terzian et al., 2012); and one took place in Washington, DC (Castel et al., 2012). What all of these studies had in common was the use of community viral load as an indicator for decreases in new HIV incidences. The rationale was that by increasing viral load surveillance, one could better understand trends in new HIV incidences. This led to an increase in 'test and treat' initiatives. The use of CVL is, as such, also aligned with the 90-90-90 targets and could indeed be read as one of many clinical implementations of the numerical targets. Another commonality between these North American studies was that they all produced maps and information based on geographical information such as postal codes as a way of visualizing their findings. In the Vancouver study, the authors stated that 'in some postal areas of the province [British Columbia], however, the proportions of potentially infectious individuals remain high regardless of the expansion of testing and treatment coverage' (cited in Gagnon & Guta, 2012b:473).

In the San Francisco study, the authors also relied on the same spatialization and visualization of CVL; two maps were produced over the city of San Francisco marking one for mean viral load and the other for total viral load (Das et al., 2010). Areas such as the Mission and the Castro were marked in mid-level blue tones indicating mean viral load metrics of under 23,348 copies/mL, the San Francisco mean (Das et al., 2010:5). However, both areas were shaded dark blue on total viral load indicating a high total viral load of above 12 million copies/mL (Das et al., 2010:5). The highest mean CVL was denoted in the Bayview area of San Francisco which on the maps was highlighted dark blue indicating a mean CVL of above 30,000 copies/mL (Das et al., 2010:5). It is interesting that the map legend also denotes Bayview and its dark blue color as 'homeless', thus signaling the low rates of viral suppression amongst homeless people living in San Francisco. Figure 3.1

The study also broke CVL up into other identity categories by presenting results on both mean CVL and total CVL for various racial backgrounds (African Americans and Latinos had the highest mean CVL among racial groups), sexual identity (transgender individuals had the highest mean CVL of all groups, while MSM had the lowest mean CVL) and intravenous drug use (IDU users had a higher CVL than the city mean) (Das et al., 2010:3). The results and subsequent recommendations made by the authors was that through CVL, public health officials could better identify 'hotspots' or areas with particular high risk of HIV infections due to the distribution of community viral load (Das et al., 2010). This, in turn, would mean that by identifying hotspots, health programs could do more community-level interventions and that more aggressive prevention efforts could be targeted more specifically (Gagnon & Guta, 2012b:474). The focus on hotspots is telling. The San Francisco study was published in 2010, and, as CVL and viral load maps have increased in usage as a surveillance method in the name of ending AIDS through geo-targeted, community-level prevention initiatives, the notion of the 'hotspot' has found its way into the new White House strategy to end AIDS by 2030. The initiative, named *Ending the HIV Epidemic. A Plan for America*, has a highly spatial focus as well as a temporal one. One of the main pillars of the strategy is a clear geographical one. The plan states that phase one will focus on geographical 'hotspots', since

> most new HIV infections in the United States are highly concentrated in certain geographic hotspots. More than 50 percent of new HIV diagnoses in 2016 and 2017 occurred in 48 counties, Washington, DC, and San Juan, Puerto Rico. We also know that seven states have a disproportionate occurrence of HIV in rural areas.
>
> (HIV.gov, 2019)

Ending AIDS, it seems, is now conceived as having its own spatio-temporal logic wherein temporality matters (ending AIDS within a set time frame, reaching certain metrics within certain times, synchronizing certain efforts by certain deadlines, etc.). However, the end of AIDS is also spatiality configured through a

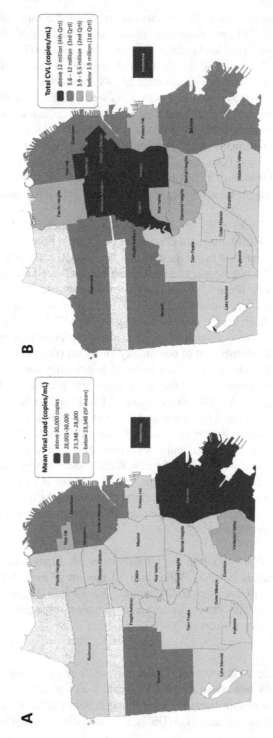

Figure 3.1 Community viral load map of San Francisco, taken from Das et al., 2010

focus on hotspots, which are then visualized through various mapping techniques meant to visualize various aspects such as CVL or new HIV infections or even prevalence. Hotspots has become a concept of significant value and concern. This new push to end AIDS through increased surveillance and testing initiatives in so-called 'hotspots', can be seen as what van Loon called 'epistemic politics' which is mainly framed within the wider logic of modern medical science, whose 'will to know' is directly coupled with the biopolitics of individual bodies and populations (Loon, 2005:46). Furthermore, hotspots exemplify how mapping of epidemic space is not only concerned with tracing the origin of a disease, mapping its trajectory or explaining its patters and regularities; as a techno-science, this mapping technique also feeds into public health management and transforms epidemic spaces into a space of 'risk flows' (Loon, 2005:46). This can clearly be envisioned in the construction of certain areas as 'hotspots' where there is a dual construction of space taking place. On the one hand, mapping constructs a space wherein public health initiatives need to be implemented with greater effort, strength and speed. On the other hand, it also constructs a space which is 'high risk', where individuals need to take precautions and where risk flows *differently* than in other spaces.

Viral load mapping and community viral loads are part of the newfound emphasis that I described in Chapter 2 on the emergence of targeted and strategic HIV efforts. The argument is that community viral load mapping can offer a form of technology that will be able to precisely monitor, locate and target communities wherein viral load numbers are higher than others places. This would allow, in theory, for the establishment of more HIV and sexual health clinics within 'hotspot' spaces, more funds going into these spaces and more community outreach programs aimed at these spaces.

However, what these maps say less about are the many intersecting dynamics that drive HIV transmissions onward and the reasons for falling out of care, thus hindering viral load suppression. Furthermore, as some activists and clinicians have pointed out, focusing solely on viral load suppression both at the community level and at the individual level reduces not only the complexities of HIV treatment but indeed reduces the nuances, needs and diversity of both individuals and communities living with HIV (Bereczky, 2019). Since viral load mapping is solely in the business of mapping and monitoring viral loads, complexities are reduced. Even with the combination of epidemiological data on income levels and stratified by racial backgrounds, the usage of viral load maps seems to offer a static understanding not only of how transmissions happen but also of what constitutes 'successful' living with HIV at the community level. Access to ARVs and achieving suppressed viral load numbers is, of course, a truly remarkable event in the history of HIV. The science behind 'undetectable = untransmissable' is undeniable and unbelievable in many ways. Yet, a sole focus on this seems to belie that 'targeted and strategic' efforts meant to lower viral loads must also include housing for homeless individuals; access to holistic health care; removal of structural barriers such as HIV criminalization, discrimination (such as transphobia), racism and homophobia; and, finally, access to health care that is affordable and equitable.

Much of the same rationale can be found in both the CVL studies in Washington and New York. In the Washington study, the researchers produced two maps similar to the San Francisco study (Castel et al., 2012:351): one that represented mean CVL and another that represented total CVL. These were subsequently juxtaposed with a map showing poverty rates in the same districts and another that showed percentages of people without high school diplomas (Castel et al., 2012:351). By doing this, the authors argued that the use of CVL was a highly useful metric for measuring and predicting HIV transmissions, while also arguing for the implementation of targeted community-level HIV prevention services which take into account poverty levels and educational disparities (Gagnon & Guta, 2012b:474). However, it is worth keeping the community in mind here.

Returning to the last set of CVL studies in the North America, the New York studies were much the same as the prior studies we have looked at. In the New York studies the authors suggested that CVLs were useful to public health officials in that they offered a way of providing targeted surveillance of trends in HIV infections. Furthermore, CVLs had 'the potential to identify high risk groups and target interventions to the groups whose viral control, if achieved, will most likely result in a rapid lowering of community viral load' (Gagnon & Guta, 2012b:474). It was also noted that CVLs had the potential to 'identify groups at risk for 'sustained high viral load' such as with Bronx residents who, according to Terzian et al. (2012), are more likely to have a detectable viral load and suffer from HIV-related disparities' (Gagnon & Guta, 2012b:474). In sum, in these studies, CVL offers not only an important metric that allows for HIV surveillance at the community level, but also an important indicator which can help in targeting HIV services and uncover disparities in HIV care. While these benign and important insights that CVL offers are important, for the sake of this book, my main argument is to link CVL and the subsequent mapping with the drive to end AIDS and the effects that CVL has when linked to this discourse. That is to say that CVL might have many uses, many of them worthy of being included in the drive to end AIDS, to 'engage in discussions and debates around the use of community viral load and how it is intrinsically linked to the logics of governmentality' (Gagnon & Guta, 2012b:474). This governmentality is one of temporality and of space, responsibility and obligations as I have argued earlier.

One area of concern is that while an HIV test should always be conducted with patient informed consent, the usage of individual viral load measures in this aggregated fashion does not imply the same ethical concerns. Thus, patients' individual consent is not required in using viral load metrics in mapping HIV viral loads at the level of the 'community'. A concern with this is that these sorts of visualizations might increase stigma at the community level and frame certain neighborhoods as being 'more infectious' than others. Research has shown that on the individual level, the quest for reaching 'undetectable' seems to have created new norms for 'sero-subjectivity'; that is, people who become undetectable come to occupy a normative position of 'successful' people living with HIV, those who are able to be adherent and responsible (Cormier McSwiggin, 2017). Conversely, people who, for one reason or another, cannot achieve viral load suppression might be labeled 'irresponsible', 'infectious' and 'non-compliant' in this new sero-sta-tus landscape (Cormier McSwiggin, 2017; Persson, 2013, 2016; Race, 2001). If this is the case on the individual level, then we might ask how normativity and 'success' are measured on the communal level? How is 'success', responsibility and blame, being shifted, measured and modeled through these community viral load maps? Although these maps are mainly meant for research and public health purposes, accessing them is only a Google search away. In addition, as we shall shortly see, variations of the notion of 'geographies of risk' is already palpable in the news media.

There is another aspect of the community viral load mapping which is prob-lematic and which highlights the tension between who is present and who is absent in these maps, who is counted and who is uncounted according to Sara Davis (Davis, 2017).

An initial critique of the usefulness of viral load maps is that

> CVL will tend to underestimate the proportion of people with high viral loads in the population [...] in addition, how it translates into the actual rate of new infections (incidence) is highly dependent on the overall number of people with HIV in the population (prevalence).
>
> (W. C. Miller, Powers, Smith, & Cohen, 2013)

While this shows the potential technical shortcomings of CVLs, there is another form of shortcoming that speaks to the politics of counting. One of the main con-cerns is that CVLs must inevitably account in some way for the viral load of those who have *not been diagnosed* with HIV. Although some of the studies that have used CVL have tried to include an estimate of viral load in undiagnosed people, this is 'dependent on viral load in diagnosed people being related in some degree to viral load in the community' (W. C. Miller et al., 2013). This is highlighted by an African study 'that estimated that 38% of infections came from people who had just acquired HIV themselves' (W. C. Miller et al., 2013). This is made more problematic in that studies have shown that the people with the highest viral load in, for instance, the US might not be the ones who are undiagnosed but rather those who have been diag-nosed and then lost to care. According to the critics, CVLs have a tendency to under-estimate 'true community viral load' since they do not account for the 'uncounted' that is, both those who are yet to be diagnosed and those 'lost to care'.

Furthermore, the usage of CVLs might be complicated by the issue of preva-lence. The notion of average CVL is criticized since CVL in itself also does not mean a lot unless HIV prevalence – the proportion of people in the community with HIV – is taken into account. An example is:

> Take two populations where, in one case, 5% of people have HIV and, in the other, 0.1%. Even if the CVL of people with HIV is the same in both popula-tions, if people meet each other at random, they have 50 times more chance of encountering a person who is infectious in one community than in the other.
>
> (W. C. Miller et al., 2013)

Hence, taking into account HIV prevalence also becomes key. My point here is not to take sides in this scene of HIV science controversy; rather, I want to point out that the mapping of community viral load also circulates around the figure of the 'uncounted' the undiagnosed. This figure seems to haunt HIV science as the figure that needs to be accounted for (through modeling or statistical analysis) or found through HIV testing and enhanced surveillance efforts. Indeed, Miller et al. who provide us with a critique of the use of average CVL values still recommend a variant of this when they advocate for a method that focuses on

> the proportion of people in the whole population who have HIV viral loads above the limit of detection, or above a cutoff point, such as 1000 copies/ml. This takes HIV prevalence into account, and, because few people not in care will have low viral loads, is almost a proxy for the proportion of people in care and their retention in care.
>
> (W. C. Miller et al., 2013)

However, even this still relies on a very accurate estimate on the proportion of people living with HIV who are *not yet diagnosed*.

In the drive to end AIDS, the figure of the undiagnosed seems to haunt the maps and models used in CVL technology. Those who need to be accounted for, at the same time need to be found. Reaching the end of AIDS hinges on HIV science framing the undiagnosed as part of the calculation, yet also highlighting that there is a need to find them. Soon after the CVL research had started to take shape – and its uptake into policy not far behind – various media outlets started to produce articles on the topic. In a book that chronicles the end of AIDS, it seems natural to examine how CVL and its mapping techniques were enacted in various media forms in the US.

Viral maps and the media

One of the first websites to report on the CVL method was the US federal website, *AIDS.gov*, which is 'an official US government website managed by the US Department of Health & Human Services and supported by the Secretary's Minority AIDS Initiative Fund (SMAIF)'.[2] Its mission is to 'expand the visibility of timely and relevant federal HIV policies, programs and resources to the American public', 'to assess starting or increasing the use of new media tools by government, minority-serving organizations and other community partners to extend the reach of HIV programs to communities at greatest risk' and finally, to 'increase knowledge about HIV and access to HIV services for people most at risk for or living with HIV'.[3] HIV.gov noted in a bulletin that CVL was a public health tool that would allow public health officials to

> compare the average viral load for each of these groups [African-American women, Latino men who have sex with men, transgender women, or White injection drug users] to identify disparities across the groups. Since the goal

is for all persons who are under HIV care to have an undetectable viral load, if a neighborhood or a community or a particular group has a higher CVL, it indicates a need to intervene.

(HIV.gov, 2011)

The focus here is again on the figure of the community and the space of neighborhood; thus, it conflates space with people regarded as belonging to the same community. Identity is entangled with certain 'hotspots' and interventions are deemed necessary once CVL numbers, either mean or total are above a certain point. The cause of high CVLs is also mentioned:

> that persons are being diagnosed very late in the course of their infection, or that they are not receiving timely referral into medical care or even that they might require additional adherence counseling in order to maintain consistent ARV use.

(HIV.gov, 2011)

It is interesting to note that of these three potential causes of high VL amongst individuals, two of them can be read as directly aimed at the individual and not at systemic issues of health disparities. Late diagnosis could imply that the individual has not tested frequently enough. A reading which is less individualistic would perhaps place the onus on lack of health care services, homelessness and lack of HIV services. 'Additional adherence counseling' clearly places the onus of adherence onto the individual and suggests that only through medical counseling could this be rectified. Leaving this aspect of the ways in which CVLs are enacted through AIDS.gov, we note that the focus is once again on how CVLs are an important metrics for rectifying community HIV disparities and thus are not only of clinical value for the individual but can indeed, when clustered as a community metric, uncover and point to health disparities. This sort of rhetorical enactment is also found in other media outlets and the way they report on the use of CVLs.

An article in POZ magazine[4] online version describes how CVL in San Francisco showed how 'some areas like the Castro – the city's gay epicenter – have more HIV cases, but that individuals in low-income neighborhoods such as Potrero Hill and Bayview have the highest viral loads and are in more need of treatment' (POZ, 2009). The use of CVL here is enacted as a way of targeting some areas more than others for treatment since PLHIV who are undetectable and stable on medication pose no threat to onward transmission, whereas people in Potrero Hill and Bayview pose both a threat to themselves, their health and to onward transmission. The POZ.com article goes on to cite Dr. Grant Colfax, director of HIV prevention and research in the city's health department, who calls the map 'a thermometer' for measuring the city's HIV epidemic. '"We're taking an individual marker and making it a marker for community health", he said' (POZ, 2009). The interesting clue here is the 'transition' that viral load metrics can make from individual marker to community marker. The seamless transfer between the individual and the community through the viral load number seems to allow for endless scalability, from individual to community to nation to global and translatability; that is, no matter what scale it is found at, the viral load metrics serve as the marker for successful HIV treatment. In the POZ.com article, space is also given an important role as when Julio Montane, president of the International AIDS Society, is quoted as saying

> you can identify hot spots where, in all likelihood, most transmission is occurring [...] These hot spots are perpetuating themselves, increasing infection in marginalized communities. This is unacceptable. As long as we don't deal with that problem, the reservoir of HIV will ensure that we're promoting the continued spread of HIV in perpetuity.
>
> (POZ, 2009)

While my critique here is not aimed at the science nor at the intentions to use community viral load mapping for good use, the dogmatic focus on *only* reducing onward HIV transmission through the lowering of viral load numbers once again seems to belie the social side of the epidemic. I realize that not every research or public health official can always include statements on the social side of HIV prevention, but there is a striking divide between biomedical and social interventions. In the above quote, the notion that 'these hotspots' are 'perpetuating themselves' is important, yet the question of *why* they are perpetuating themselves is left unanswered or at least partly unanswered. Viral load maps might be able to tell us some of the dynamics of HIV epidemics, but its not the whole story, nor should it be the sole story.

Hotspots become spaces of infection, space is invoked as a space of potential risk and the mapping of these hotspots becomes key in ending AIDS and, implicitly at least, getting rid of the hidden 'reservoir' of HIV. In perhaps a too metaphorical reading of Montane, his usage of the 'reservoir' as being place bound seems uncannily close to the very fact that the HIV virus itself indeed lays within dormant reservoirs within the body of people living with HIV. Without taking this metaphorical reading too far, it is worth noting that one of the main issues with modern day HIV treatment is that HIV 'latent reservoirs', as they are called, are hard to reach by modern day ARVs. In fact, latent HIV reservoirs are a 'group of immune cells in the body that are infected with HIV but are not actively producing new HIV [...] Finding ways to target and destroy latent reservoirs is a major challenge facing HIV researchers. Researchers are exploring different strategies for clearing out reservoirs'.[5] In a metaphorical irony, space, both corporal and geographical, becomes a site of surveillance and intervention. Both the latent, infected CD4+ T cell reservoirs and various urban hotspots become spaces of concern, interventions and surveillance. Space it seems, like time, becomes problematized in ways that allow for interventions in various shapes and forms, predicated upon rationales which are often seen as benign; yet, as I have argued, we need to attend to some of the ways in which these mappings, these spaces and these interventions might have unintended consequences. It is to some of these that I now turn.

Spaces of risk: viral load maps and the governmentality of the end of AIDS

There are two distinct entities that emerge through the above breakdown of the epistemology of CVLs as they figure in HIV prevention: one is the production of particular spaces, and the other is the production of a particular figure, the community. Let us start with the production of space. Space in the logic of the CVL is produced through a continuum of low to very high viral load numbers, either calculated as a mean or as a totality. This production of space can be linked to the work of Foucault and his notion of governmentality and security (Foucault, 2007). Foucault's shift in the geography of space in relation to infectious disease can be seen in his delineation from leper colony to plague city, in which space is produced differently in the two modalities (Foucault, 1990). In the leper colony, total seclusion and quarantine is offered, while, in the plague city, segmentation within the city is now the norm. His notion of the interplay between disciplinary actions to contain infectious disease and his term of securitization are useful for us in looking at the spaces that CVLs produce. Disciplinary governmental initiatives of space involve clear demarcations such as walls, the construction of clearly segmented parts of the city and the clear areas of access defined by clear orders of social hierarchy; in short, discipline belongs to the order of construction (Foucault, 2007:17). Disciplinary techniques of space thus include those architectures of space (in the broad sense) in which the individual is subjected to 'a series of adjacent, detective, medical and psychological techniques appear which fall within the domain of surveillance, diagnosis, and the possible transformation of individuals'(Foucault, 2007:5). In relation to infectious diseases, a clear example of the disciplinary architecture and construction of the city would be areas of quarantine of people who are sick. In fact, Lakoff contrasts discipline with security by saying that 'If disciplinary mechanisms seek to restrict the circulation of disease, isolating the sick from the healthy – as in quarantine – security mechanisms allow disease to circulate but minimize its damage through collective interventions such as mass vaccination' (Lakoff, 2015:42). At the time of writing this book, the emergence of the novel Coronavirus (nCoV) in the Hubei region in China, can illustrate Lakoff's take of Foucault. The nCoV virus causes, in certain cases, severe respiratory symptoms, which in many cases has led to hospitalization and, in some cases, death. The outbreak was declared a 'public health emergency of international concern (PHEIC) on 30 January 2020'.[6] Contrasting the nCoV outbreak with the usage of CVL in the HIV efforts clearly demonstrates the security dimension of HIV response while also highlighting the disciplinary response to nCoV. Case in point is the mass quarantine of people as China locked down a dozen cities, amounting to some 50 million people in quarantine within the cities they live and barring travel in or out of the cities[7]. Chinese authorities implemented quarantine on a scale never seen and, in response to the outbreak of nCoV, implemented drone surveillance as a tool for making sure people adhered to the quarantine parameters.[8] Clearly, the Chinese response is more in line with the disciplinary frameworks that Foucault described than they are a form of securitization of nCoV.

As such, CVLs can be seen as being part and parcel of a surveillance not of disciplinarity, but of security; that is, it maps in a dual fashion both the geographical space of the city, but by juxtaposing this with the inner space of the bodies of PLHIV, and creates a topography wherein geographical space is overlaid with a viral topography. In a health prevention context, a disciplinary strategy would seek to eradicate an infectious disease by employing techniques like arrest, quarantine and isolation, while security calculations would take the acceptable level of incidences into account, or in this case, the acceptable CVL, and weigh the costs of intervention against the risks of allowing the disease to circulate.

CVLs do not profess to create a space of quarantine, rather CVLs produce a space of security wherein what is monitored are two dual spaces; one is the concrete space of urban neighborhoods and the other space is the interiority of the bodies of various 'communities'. Moreover, since CVLs do not provide maps meant to quarantine bodies, CVL mapping produces a map over the circulation of bodies and viruses. CVL mapping techniques can be seen as being in the business of monitoring circulation and not containment per se. Since CVLs' main preoccupation is to monitor where the virus is *most likely to circulate*, CVL mapping techniques deal with minimizing circulation of the virus through the mapping of *where* it is most likely to be transmitted onward, that is, where it *will* be circulating.

This is perhaps why the authors of several of these studies focus more on the mean CVL than the total CVL, as a high mean CVL could indicate poor viral load suppression while a high total viral load count could mean either (i) some people are unsuppressed with high VLs or (ii) a great number of people living with HIV who are virally suppressed (Das et al., 2010). This was the case in the San Francisco study wherein the authors found a high *total* CVL but a low mean CVL amongst people living in the Castro area of the city. This indicated a high number of PLHIV who were virally suppressed.

While discipline strives for perfection, eliminating the abnormal or unwanted, security instead operates with levels of acceptability. Hence, security 'establishes an average considered as optimal on the one hand, and, on the other, a bandwidth of the acceptable that must not be exceeded' (Foucault, 2007:6). This can clearly be seen in the various CVL maps wherein a mean is established for the entire city and thus made into the norm for CVLs (Castel et al., 2012; Das et al., 2010). Reading Foucault into the context of CVL maps, we might say that the 'optimal' is the production of a CVL across the entire grid of measurement in the city of an 'undetectable' CVL, while the 'bandwidth of the acceptable' is the realization that some might never reach undetectable levels of viral load.

This also shows that CVLs, as a mapping technique which contributes to the securitization of the end of AIDS is highly statistical in nature, are bound to the time-space of viral load measurement intervals provided by public health authorities. This also points to the biopolitical nature of CVL, wherein despite the more tempered aspirations of security vis-a-vis disciplinary containment techniques, one still requires statistical knowledge of disease patterns to plan and measure securitization efforts to contain disease. For example, data on the mean and total

CVL of HIV viremia within an exposed population can inform efforts to lower the infection risks posed by certain practices, which of course is the rationale of the proponents of CVLs as a way of ending AIDS.

Now the spaces created through the CVLs also have another function in that they produce spaces open to being governed in a specific way. As we have seen, one of the main arguments for the use of CVLs as part of the ending of AIDS is that CVLs have the ability to zoom in on particular areas which are disproportion-ally affected by high CVLs and thus CVLs can contribute to targeted and intensi-fied public health interventions, be that scale-up of HIV testing services, scale-up of adherence programs or access to ARVs. As Guta and Gagnon states:

> what is important is not just that these spaces are rendered visible through viral load mapping and thus governable, but the particular ways in which they are constructed base on the average viral load burden of populations who occupy them and the absolute level of virus that circulates among them.
>
> (Gagnon & Guta, 2012b:475)

Gagnon and Guta build on Huxley and his tri-part division of spatial rational-ity when they analyze viral load mapping. It is worth including here some of Huxley's thinking in our own analysis.

Huxley conceptualizes three ways in which space is governed: dispositional, generative and vitalist (Huxley, 2006). The two of interest for us in this context are the dispositional and the generative. Dispositional spatial rationality, Huxley states, is a 'spatial rationality aiming at drawing boundaries and producing order that will foster correct comportments. It operates with the logics of grids of classification for the spatial disposition of "men and things", to bring arrange-ment and visibility to bear on individuals and populations' (Huxley, 2006:774). Furthermore, dispositional spatial rationality is a form of spatial rationality, which is concerned with

> spaces of debauchery, drunkenness, idleness that produce poverty, disease and death. It is bodies and behaviours out of control in unruly places, threatening to expand and spread throughout the whole city or society. This problem is the object of 'police' and 'disciplinary' constructions of spaces that will ena-ble surveillance and control of bodies and comportments. Simultaneously, however, dispositional logic also aspires to produce 'eutaxic' (well-ordered) spaces.
>
> (Huxley, 2006:775)

Read in relation to CVL mapping techniques, dispositional spatial rationalities are clearly seen in the work of CVL mapping to arrange space according to a continuum of metric values, means and totals. Cities, such as San Francisco and Washington, are spatiality arranged according to a grid of viral metrics and then shaded in color going from lighter colors, indicating low viral loads, to darker colors, indicating high viral loads. It brings to bear the visibility of 'men and viruses' as much as 'men and things' and orders space according to neat districts according to CVL metrics. Of course, what this kind of spatial logic and ordering of space cannot capture is the networks, mobility and interconnectedness of human networks be they sexual, social, or economical. The challenge of mobility to CVL has in fact been challenged by other medical geographers who have cast doubt on the feasibility of reaching the 90-90-90 targets due to the fact that people are mobile and, as such, so is the HIV virus. The CVL logic of spatialization seems to be unable to account for this and visualizes the world as a static space wherein the city is neatly divided into spaces ranging from low to high CVLs. To end AIDS within this rationality is to end it within a static understanding of *where* HIV is, not how it moves. This can be captured well in a recent map published in 2016 by the website *GetTested.com* which was an at-home STI testing company. The map, represented by the online news site, *South Florida Gay News* and on the NATAP (National AIDS Treatment Advocacy Project) website,[9] is of the entire USA with all the states shaded in colors ranging from grey, to teal, to green and then blue, where grey indicates low risk and blue indicates high risk. The map also lists 'America's riskiest cities for HIV', with Baton Rouge, Louisiana topping the list with 44.7 new HIV infections per 100,000.[10] The map's text reads 'Where you live can impact your risk of becoming infected with HIV' and then it urges people to get tested.

The point of this example, in combination with the CVLs seen earlier, is that risk of infection based on spatial logics of viral loads or prevalence produces spaces of risk. However, these spaces are reproduced as being static spaces of risk, ordered through the dispositional logic akin to the one outlined by Huxley. Mobility is not taken into account in these maps, and thus, risk is embedded into the ground so to speak, with place taking precedence over mobility and circulation.

This is not to say that there are no maps that track HIV infections through time *and* space. In fact, modern epidemiology oftentimes uses so-called 'sexual network maps' and the tracing of 'index cases' made particularly (in)famous in the HIV epidemic through the search for 'patient zero' (McKay, 2017; Pépin, 2013). Epidemic space, as van Loon calls it, has always focused on temporality as well as space; through 'a focus on disease vectors, one is able to map the complex connectivity of epidemic space, which involves a tracing of origins, causes and effects over time (Loon, 2005:45). This has certainly been the case with the HIV epidemic, wherein maps have sought to chart both the global spread of the HIV as envisioned by several maps portrayed in the media.

The second spatial logic of use is what Huxley calls 'generative rationality' (Huxley, 2006:777). For Huxley generative rationality represents a form of spatial rationality that draws on 'medico-biological conceptions of the environmental generation of disease and moral decay [...] That is, the qualities of environments are held to be catalysts in generating disease or health, immorality or virtue' (Huxley, 2006:777). The issues of the spatial rationality in this frame is not so much the disposition of spaces but rather the concentration of diseased bodies in a geographical area (Gagnon & Guta, 2012b:476). CVL mapping and its subsequent focus on the concentration of viral load metrics, such as mean and total

CVL, are examples of this. Within this rationality, the focus is moved from the disposition of diseased bodies in space and onto areas where the disease is highly concentrated and thus where the risk of transmission is intensified (Gagnon & Guta, 2012b:476). This can clearly be seen if we recall the prior studies and media concern that CVLs and their mapping is meant to specifically target certain areas of high CVL and that CVLs offer a way of responding to the 'problem' of HIV and its spread within urban settings. The use of CVL mapping can thus be seen within the framework of securitization of HIV prevention as well as part of a generative spatial rationality. Within the aforementioned CVL studies and their media enactments, CVLs are framed as being able to shift the focus away from a general HIV prevention, which is not targeted, and more toward specific areas which are deemed as vulnerable and in need of intervention and attention.

Another issue is the way in which these maps offer a certain set of associations linked to the areas wherein CVLs are higher than others. There is a duality in the usage of CVL and the mapping of this. On the one hand, CVL is highlighted as being a valuable tool in 'understanding HIV where you live' as proclaimed by AIDSVu.org (AIDSVu, 2020). This is also highlighted by the various authors of CVL research articles as well as public health officials who underscore the usefulness of CVL maps in pointing out 'vulnerable communities' and CVLs' potential to target interventions where they are most needed. On the other hand, maps and headlines, as the one described by *GetTested.com*, highlight 'America's riskiest places for HIV'. In the first instance, we see the contours of CVL and maps as offering an overview of 'communities *at risk*' while in the second framing, *areas of risk* could easily become *communities not at risk, but rather, communities of risk*. Van Loon has stated that

> the infectious body is seen as ambivalent – both *at risk* and *a risk*. This ambivalence is highlighted in the organization of the modern hospital, which 'processes' at once risky and at-risk bodies, in a complex dualism of 'isolation' (sterilization) and 'care'. The infectious body, however, is never seen as discrete, but always 'open'.
>
> (Loon, 2005:43)

Paraphrasing van Loon, may we say that spaces embedded within the CVLs' topography are both *at risk* and *a risk*, and that there is a duality wherein the spaces with high mean CVLs are in need of both intensified surveillance efforts as well as care? This seems to be the rhetorical outcome if we read the various CVL scholarship in combination with how risk is connected to place and space in the media.

The usage of CVLs and mapping techniques offers what Guta and Gagnon states are a

> partial and incomplete portrait of the HIV epidemic and continues to ignore the effect of context on HIV vulnerabilities – how the virus moves within a population and how it circulates across specific networks. What it does, however, is provide the necessary arguments to intensify surveillance, testing and

prevention efforts in areas where we can find a number of people living with
HIV whose viral load is 'unsuppressed'.

(Gagnon & Guta, 2012b:476)

Guta and Gagnon's point is important. Not only can viral load maps fail to capture the complete community viral load of an area due to the failure to calculate
or know the viral load of the undiagnosed or those outside of care, but the maps
fail to provide any meaningful understanding of transmission dynamics. Gagnon
and Guta's formulation of 'partial and incomplete portrait' seems apt in this context; indeed, the play here on 'context' is also part of my point. While the maps
can offer some aggregated data on geographical viral load measures as well as
tentatively try to describe the association between communal levels of viremia
and new incidences, they cannot say anything about the *contextual* mechanism of
either the association between communal viral load measures and new cases of
HIV nor, for that matter, why levels rise or fall.

In drawing our attention to this, Gagnon and Guta highlight an important new
feature of the HIV epidemic and the growing biomedicalization of it: namely, the
introduction of a new set of binaries within the epidemic. In the early days of the
epidemic, the binary between positive/negative was for a long time one of the defin-
ing binaries, which of course as several scholars have pointed out, was further
subdivided into 'pure/dirty', 'dangerous/safe', 'promiscuous/pious', 'gay/straight'
and 'guilty/innocent' (Epstein, 1996; Farmer, 2006; Treichler, 1999). However, as
Gagnon and Guta point to, and as several ethnographic reports now show, a new
dichotomy is slowly emerging, one which is based upon the foundational binary
between 'detectable/non-detectable'. This new binary produces, as the ethnography
of McSwiggin and others show, a further division between those who achieve long
term viral suppression and those who do not. Here, notions of 'the good patient'
emerge wherein those who achieve long term viral suppression are seen as 'adherent, responsible, and rational', while those who do not are seen as 'irrational,
bad patients who are non-adherent' (Cormier McSwiggin, 2017; Persson, 2011;
Persson, Newman, & Ellard, 2017; Sangaramoorthy, 2014). CVL mapping can be
read within the same analytical lens: on the one hand, it is clear that CVL mapping
can be a useful tool in the drive to end AIDS, but this presupposes a political will
to engage with the many syndemic factors that facilitate the HIV epidemic and not
just a narrow biomedical approach to achieve viral suppression; on the other hand,
in an era wherein these viral load maps and other HIV mapping tools are readily
available to the public, it is paramount that the ways in which notions of risk and the
spatialization of the epidemic down to local postal codes is communicated in such a
way that PLHIV in these areas are not further stigmatized.

Ending (community) AIDS? Communities at risk
and the governmental logic of surveillance

Analyzing CVL maps and other maps which are currently circulating within the
discourse of ending AIDS offers us a way of looking at how various spaces are

being created discursively in policies and in public health initiatives. Following Carol Bacchi's work, we might pause and question how certain places become specific 'objects' of importance within policy formation (Bacchi & Goodwin, 2016:96). In relation to CVL and HIV maps, we have previously looked at how certain areas become spaces of risk and infection, but also how they are high-lighted as spaces in need of care, strategic interventions and increased HIV fund-ing. As such, the 'inscription' of these spaces in policy, through CVL mapping, should be critically investigated in terms of the ways in which these spaces are being 'made' or *come to be* inscribed as specific spaces in need of surveillance.

However, the focus on CVL maps and subsequent spatialization of CVL across neighborhoods also inevitably produces certain 'populations' or, more precisely, different communities who are at risk. As I mentioned earlier, one of the discur-sive figures that emerges in these maps and the policies and discourse around CVL is the figure of the community. If Michel Foucault formed an important theorization of the shift from the government of the territory to the government and 'discovery' of the figure of the population (Foucault, 1990, 2007), then Peter Miller and Nikolas Rose expanded on this work by moving the focus onto the figure of the community (P. Miller & Rose, 2008). For Miller and Rose, the intro-duction of the figure of the community is distinct from the figure of the population as community engenders a new territory for the administration of collective life (Gagnon & Guta, 2012b:476). This new territory which is associated with the figure of the community has several differences compared to Foucault's notion of population.

First of all, the introduction of community allows for the re-configuration of space, that is, from a single, collective space of the population to different and discrete communities which can be located geographically or constructed virtu-ally, such as lifestyle communities, moral communities, activist communities, etc. (P. Miller & Rose, 2008:90).

Secondly, the figure of the community introduces a new collective, which can speak, act and leverage power. Communities operate through personal allegiances and active responsibilities (P. Miller & Rose, 2008:90), which means that the figure of the community makes use of specific ties, real or virtual, between indi-viduals and groups to regulate, mobilize and form politics, actions and meanings. The introduction of communities contrary to the figure of the population allows for a heterogeneity to be introduced into the figure of the population which leads to individuals being able to claim allegiances and obligations toward a community consisting of people 'imagined' to be similar to the individual (Anderson, 2006; P. Miller & Rose, 2008:105).

Thirdly, the figure of the community allows identification of individuals as members of particular communities and this, in turn, requires work to make the individuals aware of their community belonging (Gagnon & Guta, 2012b:477). This sort of work is conducted through state actions, such as census taking or map making and other activities as Benedict Anderson made so famous in his book *Imagined Communities* (Anderson, 2006). However, other forms of community making is conducted through organizational work such as political parties, NGOs and special interest organizations. Here, communities such as disability communities, gay communities, ethnic communities, religious communities and, of course, the AIDS community come to mind. Each of these creates a sense of community by the promotion of the work of educators, campaigns, activist activities and the use of symbols and narratives (P. Miller & Rose, 2008:92). This is particularly important in the context of CVL mapping and the end of AIDS narrative: Miller and Rose go on to say that various strategies for making individuals aware of their community allegiances are through efforts to raise awareness, educate, communicate and ensure that individuals come to identify with their respective community (P. Miller & Rose, 2008). The formation of communities offers a new way of both governing oneself, and a new way for others to govern communities. Community formation offers a new way of governing oneself according to the allegiances and obligations one has toward the community one belongs to; the individual governs him/herself in line with the values, goals, norms and political strategies of the community. Affiliation to communities creates new relations of identification and also new relations of mutual obligations (P. Miller & Rose, 2008:88). On the other hand, the creation of communities also allows for governments and other institutions to either ally themselves with them or oppose them. Furthermore, the figure of the community also introduces a new social body to be targeted by various sets of governmental strategies for governing these new communities. It allows for targeted governmental strategies that superficially govern specific communities. This is the dual nature of community as a figure of political actions: on the one hand, various communities lobby and work for their respective voices to be heard, their perspectives to be taken into account and for their communities to be seen (the metaphor of being seen is key here in relation to CVLs and mapping); on the other hand, while governmental logic of rule can stand in contrast to various communities and their political agendas, the figure of the community nevertheless allows governmental agencies to target specific communities with specific policies, rules and regulations. These can be benign or sinister; the point is that with the introduction of the figure of the community, a tension is born between the community in question, the individual and the state.

Let us now look at how the figure of community emerges in the workings of the mapping of *community* viral loads. As Guta and Gagnon state, community viral load is not just a means of identification or affiliation, rather, it is also used to govern individuals who are located here and not there, and whose distribution spatially often correlates with other characteristics that make them part of so-called 'risk communities' (viral load numbers, serostatus, gender, ethnicity, socio-economic status, sexuality, etc.) (Gagnon & Guta, 2012b:477). Within these forms of communities and the government of them, a focus on experts and expertise as a form of governmentality of the 'conduct of conduct' has emerged according to Miller and Rose (P. Miller & Rose, 2008:106). Governing communities in this fashion implies that members of these communities are the subject of expertise which now 'focuses on conduct itself and the cognitive and moral organization of perception, intention, action and evaluation' (P. Miller & Rose, 2008:106).

Part of this ecology of various forms of governing through communities as both a government of the self and of others, has been the establishment of a discourse of 'empowerment'. Empowerment as part of the governmentality of communities but also paradoxically, as part of emancipation as seen by some, is a 'matter of experts teaching communities, according to certain prescribed codes of active personal responsibility and moral obligations' (P. Miller & Rose, 2008:106).

Case in point: in an article published by the website *AIDSMAP*, Gesine Meyer-Rath stated that community viral maps could 'be used by activists and members of affected communities, to demand services where they really are needed' (Pebody, 2016). Empowerment here comes from access to data and CVL maps which can be used as evidence to point out disparities within the HIV epidemic and thus also highlight where resources need to be spent and on what areas and communities. This is highlighted in several of the CVL studies as well. Das et al. state that 'mapping the spatial distribution of CVL may delineate disparities, new "hotspots" or areas with particularly high HIV incidence, allowing a rapid response to target resources and interventions to populations at greatest risk' (Das et al., 2010:8). The same is echoed by Castel et al. who state that CVL mapping may also be a valuable tool in 'targeted public health interventions and treatment services to disproportionally affected areas and populations with the goals of reducing disparities in HIV prevention, care access and treatment utilization among these populations with the highest viral load burden'(Castel et al., 2012:352). Of course, the very fact that medical experts see CVL mapping as a tool for empowerment presupposes, as Miller and Rose have argued, that affected communities also inhabit expert patients, or 'lay experts', who can access these maps and utilize them in leveraging political power and highlight the disparities themselves. If not, empowerment through CVL mapping is nothing more than another set of public health initiatives that are reserved for health officials, policy makers and researchers. However, as I have highlighted before, these maps and the news about them have already become disseminated across a vast array of internet websites catering to both PLHIV, gay communities and other media outlets. In doing so, we must suspect that CVL and the subsequent mapping of CVL markers is, if not common knowledge, then knowledge that is accessible and usable for various communities. The question is how they are used and accessed by researchers, policy makers and affected communities.

Pivoting back to the formation and figuration of community as it appears in the various material on CVL mapping, we can note that much of the focus on community within the HIV epidemic in for instance the US, has been on community as a unit of identity; responsibilization of people who reside in certain neighborhoods; the empowerment of individuals located at the margins; and the expert management and outreach in risk communities (Gagnon & Guta, 2012b:478). The following quote by former US Surgeon General David Satcher in the much-lauded document, *Surgeon General's Call to Action to Promote Sexual Health and Responsible Sexual Behavior* from 2001 (Satcher, 2001), is the very definition of the responsibilization of HIV communities:

I would like to add a few words for the many thousands of persons living with HIV/AIDS in this country. We realize that you are not the enemy; that the enemy in this epidemic is the virus, not those who are infected with it. You need our support and encouragement. At the same time, it is also important that you realize you have an opportunity to partner with us in stemming the spread of this illness; to be responsible in your own behavior and to help others become aware of the need for responsible behavior in their sexual lives. Working together, we can make a difference.

(Satcher, 2001:ii)

In the above, there is a call to demarcation between at least two communities, PLHIV and those who do not live with HIV. Satcher, through a reference to partnership, highlights the point that Guta and Gagnon have made: to govern through the figure of community allows for the distribution of various degrees of responsibility, and, in this case, PLHIV are made particularly responsible for the 'stemming of' HIV. At the same time, Satcher also mobilizes HIV-affected communities as sort of 'partners', in that communities affected by HIV are to be encouraged to educate others of the need to be responsible in stopping HIV. If read in bad faith, one might argue that affected communities in this setting are doubly made responsible – both for their own behavior and that of others.

While this might be a very clear example of how we might see the responsibilization of communities affected by HIV, CVL maps and the way that community emerges in these maps and the text that follows them are also filled with aspects of responsibility, identity and, to a certain degree, empowerment. There is a duality at play in the way that the figure of community emerges in these maps and texts which also is key in understanding that CVL mapping and GIS technologies are increasingly viewed as a way of ending AIDS.

An interesting aspect of the mapping of CVL is that through the very mapping of CVL and subsequent communities that live in various areas, public health initiatives suddenly also find themselves increasingly interested in *some communities more than others*. Through tropes of 'high impact prevention', most research papers and public discourse on the topic can be seen as shifting their focus to the areas with the highest CVL. As the US Center for Disease Control has stated, 'high impact HIV prevention' involves 'cost-effective, proven, and scalable interventions that are targeted to specific populations based on disease burden [and] targeted to the right populations in the right geographic areas' (CDC, 2011). Community and space become crucial figures from where policy makers, health care officials and affected communities can rally around either to highlight disparities, target new interventions, call for increased HIV surveillance or even redirect funding from a general and holistic HIV preventive scheme to a more focused, community-based scheme. In fact, in the aforementioned AIDSMAP article, one of the fears of CVL mapping is that the data will be used to argue for a rhetoric of 'doing more with less' since 'funders were often very interested in mapping as targeting could mean that financial resources could be used more efficiently. This could be a way of justifying spending less' (Pebody, 2016). Under the auspices of 'cost effectiveness' and 'targeted interventions', austerity policies can be rolled out under the guise of 'helping those communities most in need'. In a paradoxical fashion, ending community AIDS through CVL mapping might end up, if fears become reality, less money being distributed since the short-term goal is to lower CVL to undetectable levels. A narrow biomedical 'end point' for public health initiatives might have the unintended consequence of other syndemic drivers, that fuel the HIV epidemic within certain communities, not receiving funding since the targeted funding of interventions is meant to focus on a clinical end goal of viral suppression. Ironically, the suppression of community viral loads might suppress the focus on other syndemic factors such as poverty, drug use, stigma, racism and mental health issues in affected communities.

Notes

1 See the CDC recommendation on undetectable viral load; https://www.cdc.gov/hiv/risk/art/index.html
2 See HIV.gov; https://www.hiv.gov/
3 See https://www.hiv.gov/about-us/mission-and-team
4 Poz magazine is, according to their own webpage, 'an award-winning print and online brand for people living with and affected by HIV/AIDS. Offering unparalleled editorial excellence since 1994, POZ magazine and POZ.com are identified by our readers as their most trusted sources of information about the disease'. POZ' online magazine as well as its paper version 'reach more than 70 percent of all people living in the United States who are aware that they are HIV positive' and 'more than 125,000 copies of POZ magazine are distributed at thousands of doctors' offices and AIDS service organizations nationwide'. See the 'About Us' section; https://www.poz.com/page/about-us
5 See AIDS.info for more on latent HIV reservoirs; https://aidsinfo.nih.gov/understanding-hiv-aids/fact-sheets/19/93/what-is-a-latent-hiv-reservoir-. For a more biomedically informed discussion on this see (Archin & Margolis, 2014; Chun & Fauci, 1999)
6 See the WHO statement; https://www.who.int/news-room/detail/30-01-2020-statement-on-the-second-meeting-of-the-international-health-regulations-(2005)-emergency-committee-regarding-the-outbreak-of-novel-coronavirus-(2019-ncov)
7 See articles that have reported on the usage of quarantine; https://www.bloomberg.com/news/articles/2020-02-04/will-china-s-coronavirus-quarantine-halt-the-virus and https://www.vox.com/2020/1/28/21083742/coronavirus-quarantine-wuhan-china-photos
8 See the Bloomberg report on the usage of drones in the nCoV outbreak; https://www.bloomberg.com/news/articles/2020-02-04/drones-take-to-china-s-skies-to-fight-coronavirus-outbreak
9 See NAPAT's website and subsequent map; http://www.natap.org/
10 See NAPAT's website and subsequent map; http://www.natap.org/

References

AIDSVu. (2020). Understanding HIV Where you live. Retrieved from https://aidsvu.org/.
Anderson, B. (2006). *Imagined communities: Reflections on the origin and spread of nationalism*. London: Verso Books.
Archin, N. M., & Margolis, D. M. (2014). Emerging strategies to deplete the HIV reservoir. *Current Opinion in Infectious Diseases, 27*(1), 29.

Bacchi, C., & Goodwin, S. (2016). *Poststructural policy analysis: A guide to practice.* Berlin: Springer.

Baral, S., Rao, A., Sullivan, P., Phaswana-Mafuya, N., Diouf, D., Millett, G. … Mishra, S. (2019). The disconnect between individual-level and population-level HIV prevention benefits of antiretroviral treatment. *Lancet HIV, 6*(9), e632–e638.

Bereczky, T. (2019). U=U is a blessing: But only for patients with access to HIV treatment: An essay by Tamás Bereczky. *BMJ, 366,* l5554.

Campbell, C., Cornish, F., & Skovdal, M. (2012). Local pain, global prescriptions? Using scale to analyse the globalisation of the HIV/AIDS response. *Health and Place, 18*(3), 447–452.

Castel, A. D., Befus, M., Willis, S., Griffin, A., West, T., Hader, S., & Greenberg, A. E. (2012). Use of the community viral load as a population-based biomarker of HIV burden. *AIDS, 26*(3), 345–353.

Center for Disease Control. (2011). High-impact HIV prevention CDC's approach to reducing HIV infections in the United States. Retrieved from https://www.cdc.gov/hiv /pdf/policies_NHPC_Booklet.pdf.

Chun, T.-W., & Fauci, A. S. (1999). Latent reservoirs of HIV: Obstacles to the eradication of virus. *Proceedings of the National Academy of Sciences, 96*(20), 10958–10961.

Cormier McSwiggin, C. (2017). Moral adherence: HIV treatment, undetectability, and stigmatized viral loads among Haitians in South Florida. *Medical Anthropology, 36*(8), 1–15

Das, M., Chu, P. L., Santos, G.-M., Scheer, S., Vittinghoff, E., McFarland, W., & Colfax, G. N. J.(2010). Decreases in community viral load are accompanied by reductions in new HIV infections in San Francisco, *PloS One, 5*(6), e11068.

Davis, S. L. (2017). The uncounted: Politics of data and visibility in global health. *The International Journal of Human Rights, 21*(8), 1144–1163.

Engelmann, L. (2018). *Mapping AIDS: Visual histories of an enduring epidemic.* Cambridge: Cambridge University Press.

Epstein, S. (1996). *Impure science: AIDS, activism, and the politics of knowledge* (Vol. 7). Berkeley: University of California Press.

Farmer, P. (2006). *AIDS and accusation: Haiti and the geography of blame.* Berkeley, CA: University of California Press.

Forgione, L., & Torzian, L. (2012). Trends in community viral load, new diagnoses, and estimated incidence of HIV, New York City, 2005–2009. *Paper Presented at the 19th conference on retroviruses and opportunistic infections,* Seattle, Washington, DC.

Foucault, M. (1990). The history of sexuality: An introduction, volume I. *Translator Robert Hurley.* New York, NY: Vintage Book Company.

Foucault, M. (2007). *Security, territory, population: Lectures at the Collège de France, 1977–78.* Berlin: Springer.

Gagnon, M., & Guta, A. (2012a). Mapping community viral load and social boundaries: Geographies of stigma and exclusion. *AIDS, 26*(12), 1577–1578.

Gagnon, M., & Guta, A. (2012b). Mapping HIV community viral load: Space, power and the government of bodies. *Critical Public Health, 22*(4), 471–483.

Gagnon, M., & Guta, A. (2014). HIV viral load: A concept analysis and critique. *Research and Theory for Nursing Practice, 28*(3), 204–227.

GetTested.com. http://www.natap.org/.

Herbeck, J., & Tanser, F. J. T. L. H. (2016). Community viral load as an index of HIV transmission potential, *The Lancet HIV, 3*(4), e152–e154.

HIV.gov. (2011). Community viral load: A new way to measure our progress. Retrieved from https://www.hiv.gov/blog/community-viral-load-a-new-way-to-measure-our-progress.

HIV.gov. (2019). Ending the HIV epidemic: A plan for America. Retrieved from https://www.hiv.gov/federal-response/ending-the-hiv-epidemic/overview.

Huxley, M. (2006). Spatial rationalities: Order, environment, evolution and government. *Social and Cultural Geography, 7*(5), 771–787.

Koch, T. (2011). *Disease maps: Epidemics on the ground.* Chicago, IL: University of Chicago Press.

Koch, T., & Koch, T. (2005). *Cartographies of disease: Maps, mapping, and medicine.* Redlands, CA: Esri Press.

Krieger, N. (2003). Place, space, and health: GIS and epidemiology. *Epidemiology, 14*(4), 384–385.

Lakoff, A. (2015). Real-time biopolitics: The actuary and the sentinel in global public health. *Economy and Society, 44*(1), 40–59.

Laraque, F., Mavronicolas, H. A., Robertson, M. M., Gortakowski, H. W., & Terzian, A. S. (2013). Disparities in community viral load among HIV-infected persons in New York City. *AIDS, 27*(13), 2129–2139.

Loon, J. v (2005). Epidemic space. *Critical Public Health, 15*(1), 39–52.

Lorway, R., & Khan, S. (2014). Reassembling epidemiology: Mapping, monitoring and making-up people in the context of HIV prevention in India. *Social Science and Medicine, 112,* 51–62.

McKay, R. A. (2017). *Patient zero and the making of the AIDS epidemic.* Chicago, IL: University of Chicago Press.

Miller, P., & Rose, N. (2008). Governing the present: Administering economic, social and personal life. Cambridge: Polity.

Miller, W. C., Powers, K. A., Smith, M. K., & Cohen, M. S. (2013). Community viral load as a measure for assessment of HIV treatment as prevention. *Lancet Infectious Diseases, 13*(5), 459–464.

Montaner, J. S., Lima, V. D., Barrios, R., Yip, B., Wood, E., Kerr, T. … Daly, P. (2010). Association of highly active antiretroviral therapy coverage, population viral load, and yearly new HIV diagnoses in British Columbia, Canada: A population-based study. *Lancet, 376*(9740), 532–539.

Pebody, R. (2016). Mapping local HIV epidemics can help target resources to areas with the greatest need. Retrieved from https://www.aidsmap.com/news/jul-2016/mapping-local-hiv-epidemics-can-help-target-resources-areas-greatest-need.

Pepin, J. (2011). *The origins of AIDS.* Cambridge: Cambridge University Press.

Pépin, J. (2013). *The origins of AIDS: From patient zero to ground zero. Journal of Epidemiology and Community Health, 67*(6), 473–475.

Persson, A. (2011). HIV-negativity in serodiscordant relationships: The absence, enactment, and liminality of serostatus identity. *Medical Anthropology, 30*(6), 569–590.

Persson, A. (2013). Non/infectious corporealities: Tensions in the biomedical era of 'HIV normalisation'. *Sociology of Health and Illness, 35*(7), 1065–1079.

Persson, A. (2016). 'The world has changed': Pharmaceutical citizenship and the reimagining of serodiscordant sexuality among couples with mixed HIV status in Australia. *Sociology of Health and Illness, 38*(3), 380–395.

Persson, A., Newman, C. E., & Ellard, J. (2017). Breaking binaries? Biomedicine and serostatus borderlands among couples with mixed HIV status. *Medical Anthropology, 36*(8), 699–713.

Poon, A. F., Gustafson, R., Daly, P., Zerr, L., Demlow, S. E., Wong, J. … Moore, D. (2016). Near real-time monitoring of HIV transmission hotspots from routine HIV genotyping: An implementation case study. *Lancet HIV, 3*(5), e231–e238.

Poz Magazine. (2009). Map of viral loads in San Francisco highlights HIV treatment inequities. Retrieved from https://www.poz.com/article/map-hiv-sf-treatment-1 7539-9006.

Race, K. (2001). The undetectable crisis: Changing technologies of risk. *Sexualities, 4*(2), 167–189.

Sangaramoorthy, T. (2014). *Treating AIDS: Politics of difference, paradox of prevention.* New Brunswick: Rutgers University Press.

Satcher, D. (2001). The Surgeon General's call to action to promote sexual health and responsible sexual behavior. *American Journal of Health Education, 32*(6), 356–368.

Snow, J. A. D. T. (1855). *On the mode of communication of cholera, by John Snow, much enlarged* (2nd ed.). London: J. Churchill (London).

Tanser, F., Vandormael, A., Cuadros, D., Phillips, A. N., de Oliveira, T., Tomita, A., . . . Pillay, D. (2017). Effect of population viral load on prospective HIV incidence in a hyperendemic rural African community. *Science Translational Medicine, 9*(420), eaam8012. doi:10.1126/scitranslmed.aam8012.

Terzian, A. S., Bodach, S. D., Wiewel, E. W., Sepkowitz, K., Bernard, M.-A., Braunstein, S. L., & Shepard, C. W. (2012). Novel use of surveillance data to detect HIV-infected persons with sustained high viral load and durable virologic suppression in New York City. *Plos One, 7*(1), e29679.

Treichler, P. A. (1999). *How to have theory in an epidemic: Cultural chronicles of AIDS.* Durham: Duke University Press.

4 Molecular HIV surveillance
Issues of consent, ethics and molecular truth telling

Introduction

Targeted and strategic HIV programs are the name of the game within the PEPFAR, UNAIDS Fast Track and US *Ending the HIV Epidemic. A Plan for America* strategies. It also has taken hold within various national HIV plans wherein the focus is given to specific places, people or communities. At the intersection of this, novel HIV technologies have emerged such as the use of community viral loads (CVLs) and the subsequent mapping of them. However, perhaps the technology that best exemplifies this turn toward a strict focus on key areas and populations is the use of so-called 'molecular HIV surveillance'. Here I examine how molecular HIV surveillance emerges in the HIV scientific literature and public media discourse. The focus is on how this technology, while professing to be uniquely positioned to be an integral part of the push toward ending AIDS, nevertheless also poses and possesses inherently problematic issues.

Molecular HIV surveillance is thought of as a tool wherein the goal is to identify clusters of genetically similar viral strains in 'near real time' in the communities and areas where transmission is occurring and then intervene with what has been called 'enhanced public health approaches', which includes linking people to systems of care, treatment, testing and further diagnosis (Poon et al., 2016; Little et al., 2014).

Molecular surveillance is often framed as a tool that can reach communities 'often deemed hard to reach where outbreaks would otherwise go undocumented by authorities' (McClelland et al., 2019:1). As such, molecular surveillance has been heralded by the US Center for Disease Control (CDC) as a 'critical step toward bringing the nation closer to the goal of no new infections'.[1] The usage of molecular HIV surveillance is not confined only to the US, but is also in use in Canada (Poon et al., 2016). Studies on its usage have been conducted in Spain (González-Alba et al., 2011) and France (Wirden et al., 2019; Chaillon et al., 2017). In all of these cases, health authorities

> take aggregated data from people's HIV blood tests and compares them molecularly to identify groupings of genetically similar viruses that are connected temporally, geographically, and by stage of infection. This enables

surveillance to take place among populations [...] and in locations where HIV is being transmitted among people not well-connected to care.

(McClelland et al., 2019:2)

The CDC argues that molecular surveillance is better equipped to discover and intervene in so-called 'risk networks' wherein molecular surveillance can be used to overcome traditional barriers to disease surveillance.[2] Barriers that molecular surveillance purportedly circumvent are delays between HIV infection and diagnosis which, in turn, leads to poorer health outcomes as well as higher risk of onward HIV transmission; population mobility; and the tracking down and tracing of sexual and drug-taking partners of newly infected HIV patients (Oster et al., 2018a; Oster et al., 2018b; Oster et al., 2015).

My goal is to critically engage with how molecular HIV surveillance, a practice and technology that is portrayed as a benign public health intervention, evacuates and purifies many of the social and political contexts of HIV transmissions (McClelland et al., 2019:2). Building on the work of Guta, Gagnon and McClelland, I want to place molecular HIV surveillance in connection with the public health apparatus of 'treatment as prevention', viral load metrics and its subsequent geospatial mapping (Gagnon and Guta, 2012b; Gagnon & Guta, 2012a; Guta et al., 2016b; Guta et al., 2016a). However, I also want to extend their work by focusing on how molecular HIV surveillance, through genotypic and phenotypic testing, can be read as forms of 'molecular truth-telling' surveillance devices. This has implications not only for the ethics of consent, anonymity and criminalization which has been documented in the literature (McClelland et al., 2019; Mehta et al., 2019; Coltart et al., 2018), but also for how molecular surveillance might come to discern, through genetic surveillance of HIV, people's alleged sexuality, position in 'HIV risk networks', as well as creating new risk groups, who in turn might be subject to 'enhanced HIV surveillance and interventions'. As such, the work of Nikolas Rose is also a contribution to the emerging analysis of how medical power and surveillance have extended its reach to the scale of the molecular (Rose, 2007). Following the above trajectory, I will critically examine recent HIV science studies on the usage and rationale for implementing molecular HIV surveillance as well as engaging with public discourse on its use. After this, I will elaborate on the concept of 'molecular truth-telling' and its epistemological and ethical implications, both in terms of what it claims to be able to tell us as well as implications for issues such as consent and criminalization.

Defining molecular HIV surveillance: from clinical usage to epidemiological surveillance

Phylogenetic testing is a way of mapping the genetic makeup of HIV. By mapping the genetic material of various strains of HIV, phylogenetic testing can create an evolutionary or genealogical 'tree' of the relationship of various HIV strains. Castor et al. observe that the 'first applications of phylogenetics to the study of HIV date from the early 1990s and were aimed at inferring the origins of HIV-1 and the classification of HIV into different types (1 and 2), groups (M, N, O within HIV-1) and subtypes (A–D, F–H, and J and K within Group M of HIV-1)' (Castor et al., 2012; Huet et al., 1990). Castor et al. further state that 'today, phylogenetic analysis has become a common practice of many HIV/AIDS research programs, due mainly to the many insights these analyses can provide and the novel questions they can address over a variety of topics related to HIV biology' (Castor et al., 2012:3). The use of phylogenetic testing as a clinical tool in patient-centered care has mainly been employed to map resistance to HIV antiretroviral drugs. The rise of HIV drug resistance is an issue that both public health programs and clinical care providers must take into account. In this light, the usage of such tests can be seen as an example of 'bridging the gap' between science in laboratories and clinical application – and more generally, putting research-based knowledge into practice.

Once a person living with HIV is enrolled in care in many high-income countries a range of blood tests are taken, amongst these, a genotyping of the HIV strain that the person lives with. This test then produces, through genetic sequencing, three important things: '(1) the viral subtype, (2) the presence of drug-resistant variations and (3) phylogenetic analysis to examine how viral sequences are related' (McClelland et al., 2019:2). This latter result is not collected as part of patient care and thus extends the original clinical usage of genotypic as a way of repurposing phylogenetic testing to the realm of epidemiological surveillance.

In the practical realm of HIV surveillance, these results are held in databanks by surveillance authorities, such as the National HIV Surveillance System in the US and the BC Centre for Excellence in HIV/AIDS in Canada (McClelland et al., 2019:2). Phylogenetic analysis of genotypic data of HIV strains analyzes genetically similar groups of viremia together. However, since phylogenetic testing cannot conclusively claim the directionality of transmission, the only thing that can be established is a certain degree of genetic kinship between viral strains. This produces clusters of genetically similar HIV strains that can then be monitored as they occur and reported into the various databases in use. The CDC has stated that they are particularly interested in molecular clusters with upwards of 5 new HIV transmissions within the past 12 months with no more than 0.5% genetic difference between them (CDC, 2018). Once these transmission clusters have been detected, the CDC notes that various efforts need to be used to identify and intervene in both the molecular HIV cluster in what is called the extended 'risk networks' (CDC, 2018). Risk networks are defined as 'persons among whom HIV transmission has occurred and could be ongoing. This network includes persons who are not HIV-infected but may be at risk for infection, as well as the HIV-infected persons in the transmission cluster'.[3] After identification of a transmission cluster and its subsequent risk networks, the CDC notes that it is key to intervene in both the transmission cluster and the risk network by offering HIV testing, access to care and other preventive tools such as pre-exposure prophylaxis (PrEP).

There is one important aspect to this that I want to briefly highlight. This relates to how phylogenetic testing as a tool for HIV surveillance aligns with the strategic and targeted focus that we have seen emerge in the wake of the Fast Track strategy and the 90-90-90 targets. Molecular surveillance alleges to be able to uncover not only HIV transmissions amongst a select few people but also to map entire 'HIV transmission networks', thus also inferring larger 'risk networks'.

However, less attention has been given to what happens when a medical technology that was first used as a method for testing for HIV drug resistance is repurposed for another use? What happens when the same technology crosses from one health care regime (clinical usage) to another (public health surveillance)? These are some of the questions I want to try to highlight in the next sections of this chapter.

Molecular truth-telling: uncovering hidden risk groups, networks and desires

Here I critically engage with how there is an intense focus on what 'problems' molecular HIV surveillance is suited for in the literature. This is often done through recourse to 'what molecular surveillance can uncover', a phrasing which I will return to for its many telling implications. Recent studies have focused on how molecular HIV testing can (1) infer the role of immigration on HIV dynamics, (2) 'uncover' non-disclosed men who have sex with men and (3) create a new high-risk group by once again uncovering HIV risk and infections amongst men who identify as heterosexual but who have sex with transgender women. Finally, I will link this to the issues of consent and criminalization, building on emerging literature on the topic in connection to molecular HIV surveillance (McClelland et al., 2019; Mehta et al., 2019; Coltart et al., 2018).

Inferring the role of immigration on 'HIV dynamics': the figure of the immigrant

The idea that immigration and immigrants influence local HIV epidemic dynamics is a well-known issue in the social history of the HIV epidemic. This can be discerned in the seminal work of Paul Farmer in his book *AIDS and Accusation* (Farmer, 2006), in which Farmer traces the contours of a 'geography of blame' wherein people from Haiti were labeled as being the ones who 'introduced' HIV to the US, a perspective Farmer connects to underlying notions of Eurocentrism and a colonial legacy of racism. Much the same has been argued by Steven Epstein (Epstein, 1996), Paula Treichler (Treichler, 1999) and Thurka Sangaramoorthy (Sangaramoorthy, 2014). Others have connected this to public health policies of increased HIV testing of immigrants as well as a form of governmentality of securitization wherein HIV testing of immigrants is framed as a way of securing the national population from HIV (Ingram, 2008; Persson & Newman, 2008). Little wonder then, that molecular HIV surveillance would take this problem up as a way of arguing for how molecular HIV surveillance could be used to 'map the impact of immigration' upon local HIV dynamics.

Take, for instance, a study from Madrid, Spain, which sought to use phylogenetic testing as a tool to estimate the impact of immigration on the molecular epidemiology landscape of HIV-1 in Madrid, a large urban receptor area for many immigrants and travelers, to detect the entry of new HIV-1 variants into its population and to relate the emergence and spread of these new variants with social or risky behavior groups.

(González-Alba et al., 2011:10756)

In doing so, the study first elaborated on the genetic distribution of HIV-1 subtypes in Europe, Africa, South America and, finally, Spain. The study noted that in the local Spanish population, HIV-1 subtype B had historically been the dominant strain of HIV (González-Alba et al., 2011:10756), whereas in South America the dominate strain had been the so-called 'BF recombinant' forms, and in Africa, the genetic diversity of HIV-1 was mostly non-subtype B strains (González-Alba et al., 2011:10756).

Associations between different strains of HIV become networks of potential HIV transmissions and associations can be made between immigration and potential new subtypes of HIV that are introduced to Spain through immigration. The paper alludes to as much when it states that 'these studies are especially interesting in regions with high migration rates because they might reveal how the local epidemiology of HIV is altered by immigration' (González-Alba et al., 2011:10761). The result of the study is presented as proof that immigration and, implicitly, immigrants do alter and change the HIV-1 landscape of the HIV epidemic in Spain: for instance, the study notes that 50% of all HIV-1 patients carrying subtype C were Spaniards, whereas previous studies had shown that this subtype was mainly found in immigrants (González-Alba et al., 2011:10761). Furthermore, the study goes on to make an association between immigrants from South America, transmission of non-B variants of HIV and 'native Spaniards' by way of an association which involves 'subtype C' and 'linguistic and cultural links with the Spanish population, making them very good candidates among immigrant groups for spreading imported variants' (González-Alba et al., 2011:10761). It is interesting to note that the invocation of 'linguistic and cultural links' is used as a way of inferring how HIV is transmitted. If read in bad faith, the above seems to place responsibility on immigrants from South America as it is *their linguistic and cultural links* that make *them* better 'candidates' among all immigrants for 'spreading imported variants' of HIV. Furthermore, the finding of new subtypes of HIV within 'native Spaniards' seems to indicate that agency is located within the immigrants, they are the active vector in the transmission chain, while native Spaniards are passive and merely the targets of these transmission chains.

The general problematization of immigration is often refracted through the rationale that molecular HIV surveillance is a useful public health tool. Arguments that often arise in HIV science on molecular HIV surveillance are that it can 'estimate the impact of immigration on national and local HIV dynamics' (González-Alba et al., 2011) or how certain 'risk groups' with immigrant backgrounds contributed to 'the import of other HIV strains' (Lai et al., 2020). How various HIV sciences position molecular HIV surveillance as a *solution* to the 'problem' of immigration and HIV is often framed through recourse to 'targeted HIV preventive measures' (González-Alba et al., 2011; Dennis et al., 2015), such as linkage to care and HIV testing within 'risk networks'.

However, equally as evident is how immigrants are positioned as the *active* parts in onward HIV transmissions. In one article focusing on the role of South American transgender women and their role in HIV transmissions in Italy, the authors state that 'our results indicate that South American transgenders largely contribute to the heterogeneity of HIV-1 in our country' (Lai et al., 2020). Furthermore, the article concluded that South American transgender women 'often do not practice safe sex' and that transgender women of South American backgrounds 'could have a bridging role in the spread of HIV among both Italian MSM and heterosexuals' (Lai et al., 2020). This kind of focus on the active role of immigrant MSM and transgender women were echoed in other articles both from Spain and the US (González-Alba et al., 2011, 2013; Dennis et al., 2015). One of the sub-themes in these articles is the focus on whether immigrants contracted HIV within the countries they immigrated to or became HIV-positive in their 'home countries' and then transmitted HIV onward to their countries of immigration (Dennis et al., 2015; Lai et al., 2020).

As with most of the calls for the repurposing of phylogenetic testing as a surveillance method, many papers stipulate that the intention in detecting clusters is to offer a way of targeting specific groups with preventive programs and link people to HIV treatment and care programs. While I am not refuting the claim that this sort of targeted interventions might have a place in HIV treatment and prevention programs, my main point is that such efforts should be carefully communicated to affected communities as well as the broader public to avoid stigmatization of already vulnerable groups, such as immigrants. More generally, my point is that the repurposing or translation of phylogenetic testing as a tool for molecular HIV surveillance 'black boxes' many of the aspects that it purportedly claims to be able to uncover. In the cases above, the role of immigrant MSM and transgender women to local HIV dynamics is highlighted as being substantial. Yet, little can be discerned about the role of 'native' Spaniards, Italians or Americans in the transmission networks. Furthermore, a broad range of socioeconomic factors is left out when articles focus on the 'transmission dynamics of immigrants' and their impact on 'local HIV dynamics'.

Concerning a case from Texas, Taylor and Sapién note that in the wake of results, news headlines emerged in the local news ecology that read 'Cluster of HIV Cases Involves Hispanic Men in San Antonio', and they concluded that such headlines might have increased stigma in the community toward Hispanic and Latinx men (Taylor & Sapién, 2020:2). They conclude that while the translation of phylogenetic testing from clinical usage to molecular HIV surveillance might add a tool for targeted HIV prevention and care services, they also noted that it might indeed increase stigma in already stigmatized groups.

Another case in point is the current US President Donald Trump's statement that immigrants from Haiti 'all have AIDS' as was circulated widely in the media (Mindock, 2017). The media discourse of immigrants 'bringing AIDS' to the US, Canada or Europe is a well-known trope which shows that while phylogenetic testing as molecular surveillance can be a tool in HIV prevention and access to care, the framing of it and its usage should also be contextualized within a social and political climate wherein immigrants, in particular, have been stigmatized as 'carriers of HIV/AIDS' (Wintour, 2014; Da Silva, 2018; Tani, 2015; Tondo, 2018). This becomes heightened through recent concerns that phylogenetic data might be shared or demanded to be shared with Immigration and Customs Enforcement (ICE) or law enforcement, a concern that was raised recently by Naina Khanna, executive director of Positive Women's Network. She noted that 'in this political environment, it would be foolish to assume such data would not be used to target immigrants or other vulnerable populations' (Kempner, 2019). The same is noted by Taylor and Sapién who state that some states require sharing of public health information with law enforcement (Taylor & Sapién, 2020:3). In singling out immigrants as 'vectors' for HIV transmission and by according them a form of 'active' role in shaping 'HIV landscapes', the need to be careful in how this framing of immigrants is done becomes crucial. Translating phylogenetic HIV testing from clinical care to a tool for public health surveillance seems to also run the risk of 'losing' something in this translation. In this case, a broad range of issues is 'lost in translation' if we only look at the 'transmission networks' provided to us by molecular HIV surveillance. We risk losing sight of the many complex and entangled factors that contribute to HIV transmission if we only follow the traces left by molecular bonds that connect people.

Uncovering 'risk groups': molecular truth telling, non-disclosed men who have sex with men and heterosexual men who have sex with transgender women

The fear and the focus on men who have sex with men but do not disclose this has been a focal point within the HIV epidemic since its beginning. In particular, the focus on bisexual men as vectors of onward HIV transmissions into heterosexual communities has been a focus of biomedical epidemiology (Chow et al., 2011; Montgomery et al., 2003; Wood et al., 1993; Boulton et al., 1992). This anxiety has been heightened concerning the potential of onward transmission to the female partners of 'non-disclosed men who have sex with men' (ndMSM). In particular, scholarship has focused on how the figure of the African-American bisexual man has been made an object of pathology and danger through discourses of being 'on the down-low' (Han, 2015; Stone, 2011). Since phylogenetic testing aims to uncover 'hidden populations' wherein HIV is being transmitted, many of the articles that deal with HIV molecular surveillance which I analyzed highlighted how phylogenetic testing can uncover and make visible communities wherein HIV transmissions were ongoing, where an outbreak might be imminent and which communities were clustered together genetically, thus also inferring 'hidden transmission networks' or routes. In alluding to this, the articles also highlighted how some men who had acquired an HIV infection had done so through sex with other men and not, as they had reported, through heterosexual contact.

A case in point is the article 'Phylogenetic analyses reveal HIV-1 infections between men misclassified as heterosexual transmissions' (Hué et al., 2014). By stipulating that 'HIV-1 subtype B infections are associated with MSM in the UK. Yet, around 13% of subtype B infections are found in those reporting heterosexual contact as transmission route' (Hué et al., 2014:1967), the authors assert that public health programs can identify men who have been 'misclassified' as heterosexual risk subjects through phylogenetic testing. By using phylogenetic testing, the authors infer that they can trace, through transmission chains, HIV infections 'that may be incorrectly ascribed to heterosexual risk rather than sex between men' (Hué et al., 2014:1968). In doing so, the authors state that they are for the first time able to 'quantify nondisclosure of homosexually acquired infections reported through national surveillance and illustrate how phylogenetic inference can complement traditional epidemiological analyses' (Hué et al., 2014:1968). The study showed that 'our estimates suggest that between 1% […] and 21% of Black African men reported as heterosexual most likely acquired HIV through sex with other men' (Hué et al., 2014:1973). The authors infer this from genetic analysis of subtypes of HIV that are found in clusters of people living with HIV and then linking these with subtypes that dominate MSM communities. In doing so, an association is made and a network is being traced through the genetic family resemblance of HIV-1 viruses linking MSM and ndMSM, in particular, Black African men. Yet most of the social aspects of this network are left out of the article, and, as with many of the other networks traced, the social aspect of human sexuality and intimacy is left outside the analysis.

Most of the articles that focused on this issue highlighted the 'problem' to be solved was that men who had sex with men, but did not disclose this, posed a blind spot in HIV epidemiology (Hué et al., 2014; Ragonnet-Cronin et al., 2018). Furthermore, and most importantly, was that the 'non-disclosed men who have sex with men' were important to uncover for the potential they had in being a 'bridge' between MSM HIV dynamics and heterosexual HIV dynamics (Ragonnet-Cronin et al., 2019a). A final rationale was that molecular HIV surveillance could be used to notify men who identified as heterosexual about their risk of HIV if they had sex, for instance, with transgender women (Ragonnet-Cronin et al., 2019b). The 'uncovering of non-disclosed men who have sex with men' comes through establishing genetic kinship between strains of HIV found in clusters of men who have sex with men and then comparing this to men who do not report having sex with other men. The authors infer this from genetic analysis of subtypes of HIV, which are found in clusters of people living with HIV and then linking these with subtypes that dominate MSM communities.

Phylogenetic testing offers in this optic a way of discerning what is hidden: not only an HIV infection, its transmission networks and chains, but also how people have acquired HIV, i.e., the *type* of 'risk exposure' of heterosexual men who have sex with men. 'Male heterosexuals who have sex with men, but are not identified as "gay" are also likely to misreport their potential exposure' (Hué et al., 2014:1973). The notion that phylogenetic testing not only can trace transmission networks and transmission chains is being supplemented by its ability to discern the 'truth' about a subject's sexuality in a way that seems to circumvent the subject's reporting on the topic.

This is also be exemplified by the focus on men who identify as heterosexual but who have sex with transgender women. Here too, we find the idea that phylogenetic molecular HIV surveillance can be of use in uncovering and also *telling* people something about their risks emerges. In a review article scoping the uses of genetic HIV surveillance in 'disclosed and cryptic HIV transmission risk', the authors highlight non-disclosed MSMs as one such important vector (Ragonnet-Cronin et al., 2019a). Furthermore, the article also argues that partners of transgender women are key as they represent groups at high risk of HIV (Ragonnet-Cronin et al., 2019a:209) and that since these men often do not recognize themselves as being a distinct 'risk group', they may end up underestimating their own risk of HIV (Ragonnet-Cronin et al., 2019a:209).

In this optic, genetic HIV surveillance serves a dual purpose: first, it purportedly allows for the 'uncovering' of a new risk group, heterosexual men who do not identify as gay but have sex with transgender women; second, it also supplements these men's sense or understanding of being 'at risk'. The rationale is that genetic surveillance allows public health authorities to uncover the 'true risk' of these men since they might underestimate their HIV risk as they have not come to recognize themselves as a 'risk group'.

However, the notion that phylogenetic tests can, at the molecular level, infer if a man has had sex with another man even though he does not disclose having sex with other men poses a serious ethical issue for people who handle this data. Even researchers who argue for the usefulness and novelty of genetic HIV surveillance warn against this. As Ragonnet-Cronin notes, 'questioning heterosexual men regarding potential male partners risks alienating those men and leading to mistrust of health institutions' (Ragonnet-Cronin et al., 2019a:209). Indeed we might speculate that this sort of usage, if not handled in an ethical manner involving the affected communities, might lead non-disclosed men who have sex with men to not test or at least become hesitant toward how their results are communicated, stored and, indeed, *seen* by health care personnel. The Center for HIV Law and Policy states, building on research that mistrust might increase amongst vulnerable communities where an already existing mistrust to medical authorities is present.[4] The process of translating phylogenetic testing from clinic to surveillance seems to pose some serious ethical and epistemological questions, such as our capacity to tell the truth about our sexuality, our health and our risks.

Molecular truths, surveillance and subjectivities: speaking truthfully about sex and HIV

From a Foucauldian perspective, phylogenetic molecular surveillance seems to profess to be able to provide panoptic surveillance at the molecular level which can show us who is having sex with each other, who is not disclosing their risks and who is, perhaps, even lying. Tim Dean has argued for this in relation to how viral load measurements also provide this sort of panoptic system of surveillance for monitoring patients' adherence to their HIV medications (Dean, 2015). In monitoring active drug levels in dried blood that had been drawn from people living with HIV, clinicians can discern how adherence to the drug is followed by relying on the objective measure of active drug levels detected rather than on the reported adherence of the patient. As seen above, similar ways of surveilling on a molecular level whom people are intimate with seems to be in play. Both technologies – testing for active drug levels in the blood to monitor adherence and molecular transmission tracing – offer ways of circumventing the subject's own willingness to disclose either adherence levels or with whom they have sex. This is, in and of itself, an ethical issue that needs to be explored in more detail. It also inserts these sorts of surveillance technologies in the larger discussion on molecular biopolitics as it figures in the scholarship of Nikolas Rose (Rose, 2007; Rabinow & Rose, 2006; Rabinow & Rose, 2003). This scholarship focuses on the tension on the one hand between 'genetic risk' and genetic responsibility and, on the other, how a 'molecular optic' 'transforms the relations between patient and expert in unexpected ways and is linked to the development of novel "life strategies", involving practices of choice, enterprise, self-actualization and prudence in relation to one's genetic make-up' (Novas & Rose, 2000:1).

However, my argument is that molecular HIV surveillance is less about the optimization of life itself or health but more about an alleged optimization of the gaze of public health surveillance. Molecular HIV surveillance is a form of surveillance which extends what David Armstrong dubbed 'surveillance medicine' (Armstrong, 1995) to the scale of the molecular. Armstrong's genealogy of 'medical spaces', as Michel Foucault also worked on (Foucault, 2002), shows us how the 'clinical gaze' has transformed from what Armstrong calls 'Bedside Medicine' in the 18th century to 'Hospital Medicine' in the 19th and 20th centuries and, finally, to 'Laboratory Medicine' and 'Surveillance Medicine' in the 21st century (Armstrong, 1995:395). Each of these forms of medicine has its way of spatializing disease and illness. While space consideration forecloses a complete re-reading of Armstrong's arguments, I argue that molecular HIV surveillance now not only spatializes disease and risk onto sophisticated geospatial maps but indeed extends its mapping of medical and risk spaces into the interiority of people. Mapping is no longer only concerned with mapping disease onto maps such as in the famous epidemiological maps developed by John Snow to map cholera outbreaks in London (Snow, 1855). Now the mapping of molecular traces produces new forms of spatializing HIV through the molecular bonds that bind people who live with HIV and, thus, new notions of connectivity, networks and risk. This, I argue, is also the result of a process of translation; if translation, as it is understood within science and technology studies and actor-network theory, postulates that translation produces new associations and new connections, then molecular HIV surveillance seems to offer us a way of thinking through how new networks are being created through concepts such as 'risk networks' and 'transmission networks'. However, as I argued above, we should also try to evaluate what these concepts mask as much as what they 'uncover'. In creating new associations and new networks, molecular HIV surveillance seems also to sever or mask other aspects of HIV transmissions, such as structural drivers, cultural aspects and economic disparities.

This sort of surveillance medicine is, as Dean notes, part of the historical moment when 'biopower extended its reach inside human bodies via drugs that regulate sexuality at the molecular level' (Dean, 2015:236). Dean connects this moment to the introduction of the contraceptive birth control pill, now known only as 'the pill' and then builds on this argument to insert the introduction of PrEP against HIV as part of this movement to extend biopower to the level of the molecular. Preciado and Dean argue that 'power acts through molecules that incorporate themselves into our immune system'. Biopower gets inside us not only through psychological mechanisms of identification (as we figure out who we truly are sexually) but also through the pharmaceuticals we ingest to become the sexual beings we aspire to be.

(Preciado, cited in Dean, 2015:237)

However, I want to reverse this: rather than reading how pharmaceuticals alter our molecules for us to *become sexual citizens* or engage with sexual practices, I argue that molecular HIV surveillance reverses this and exerts biopower through its ability to infer our risks, our sexual and intimate lives through molecular bonds that bind us through the mediation of HIV viremia. Biopower in this optic is not something that *gets inside us* or that is incorporated into our immune system by way of pharmaceuticals. Rather, it is something that is *extracted and inferred* from us through molecular genotyping of HIV viremia. It is incorporated into our immune system not through pharmaceuticals but through living with HIV. Surveillance and truth-telling have become miniaturized and 'molecularized' in a way that is an extension of surveillance medicine. As Preciado notes, 'We are gradually witnessing the miniaturization, internalization, and reflexive introversion (inward coiling toward what is considered intimate, private space) of the surveillance and control mechanisms of the disciplinary sexopolitical regime' (Preciado, 2013:79). This turn toward the interiority of the subject by way of molecular HIV surveillance has consequences not only for the subjectivity of people living with HIV or at risk of HIV, but it also has potentially grave ethical ramifications having to do with stigma, consent and criminalization of HIV. It also has, as I have argued above, ethical ramifications for how we come to understand what can be said about sex and sexuality concerning the tension between the subjects' sense of risk, desire and sex and molecular HIV surveillance. These ethical issues have to do with how we can truly speak about sex and how we frame risk and responsibility. Molecular HIV surveillance offers a clear problematic space in terms of how molecular surveillance proposes to 'speak truthfully' about a person's risk, HIV transmission history, as well as how whole communities reform 'HIV landscapes'.

In translating phylogenetic testing from the clinic to the domain of epidemiological surveillance, something else entirely is being extracted from the information given by molecules in the blood of people living with HIV. No longer is the focus on extracting information about the resistance levels of the HIV strain in question; rather, what is extracted is a *trace* of who people are intimate with, whom they desire and what forms of risk they take. In the process of translating phylogenetic testing from clinical usage to epidemiological surveillance, what is extracted is not information on drug resistance; rather, the extracted information is seen as being a form of index or having a form of indexicality. By this I mean that information on genetic kinship between similar HIV strains becomes indexes for who people are intimate with, what they desire and, to a certain degree, what type of sexual identity they have (e.g., 'non-disclosed men who have sex with men', men who identify as heterosexual but have sex with transgender women).

The repurposing of phylogenetic testing from clinical usage to molecular surveillance shows us how molecular technologies, when repurposed for surveillance goals, suddenly also become technologies that can increase stigmatization through a sort of 'molecular panopticon of suspicion'. Here the subject's capacity to tell 'the truth' about desire, risk and transmission is always in danger of being overridden by the technological apparatus of molecular testing. The crossing over from clinic to surveillance seems to indicate that these HIV technologies have a common capacity or aspiration to uncover 'hidden truths' at the molecular level, discern risks that were unknown to the subjects themselves and unmask both people's sexual networks as well as their connectivity through a molecular bond.

The ethics of it all: consequences of translation

At the heart of the translation of the use of molecular HIV surveillance lies the ethical issues of consent and stigma. Whereas an HIV test always needs to be conducted with the explicit consent of the patient, the subsequent genotypic test and data material are exempt from this. Phylogenetic data are sent directly to databanks without the subject's knowledge that it is being sent. In light of the many states and nations that in some shape or form still criminalizes HIV and onward HIV transmission, this is particularly worrisome (McClelland et al., 2019). While directionality cannot be inferred by phylogenetic testing, usage of this sort of technology has been taken to court in several countries as forensic evidence (Bernard et al., 2007). However, Bernard et al. warn that such usage of surveillance data as forensic evidence for the 'reckless transmission of HIV' needs to be checked by a solid evidence base and that 'over-interpreting the results of phylogenetic analyses is unacceptable, regardless of how convinced an expert may be of the guilt or innocence of the accused' (Bernard et al., 2007:386). This highlights the dangers of misuse of phylogenetic testing as a form of forensic technology, an issue that in and of itself poses serious ethical considerations of the technology in question.

From a public health perspective, there is also the ethics of resources and the evidence that this form of surveillance is doing what it proposes to do. As McClelland et al. state: 'as of 1 January 2018, the CDC has started providing funding to all health departments for the reporting and monitoring of these results as part of efforts to expand the scale-up of molecular surveillance' (McClelland et al., 2019). Yet, the evidence base that molecular HIV surveillance is cost-effective, reduces HIV incidences and links more people to care and treatment is still uncertain. The Center for HIV Law and Policy notes: 'It is also not clear that this data, which comes from people already in care, provide uniquely useful prevention information that is otherwise unavailable' (Center for HIV Law and Policy, 2018). Naina Khanna, executive director of Positive Women's Network stated in an interview that she was critical to the notion that this sort of technology

> provides anything we don't already know or couldn't get from sitting down with a group of transgender women in Los Angeles. She worries that these analyses are becoming more common because researchers get excited about fancy new technologies and consistently undervalue old-fashioned social science research and not because the new technologies add anything of importance.
>
> (Kempner, 2019)

This also highlights the need to critically engage with what is funded and not funded and how this new form of HIV surveillance might detract funding from other more traditional public health initiatives and redirect funding to a technology whose efficacy is questionable.

The Center for HIV Law and Policy notes that the aforementioned ethical and legal issues come together at a historical moment when several other legal and policy issues are eroding the rights of people living with HIV as well as potentially heightening stigma and increasing distrust in medical institutions by vulnerable communities. These issues include 'numerous efforts to bypass basic patient protections in the name of ending the HIV epidemic, including a legislative proposal to dispense with direct notice and consent of HIV test in New York' (Schneider & Birnbaum, 2019). Furthermore, the Center for HIV Law and Policy states that many of these issues intersect at a time of at least two very worrisome trends. First is a belief that because the end of the HIV epidemic appears to be within reach any means to reach that end are justified, even if they fly in the face of medical ethics and respect for the dignity of people living with HIV and marginalized communities. Second is the mistaken perception that increased representation of people living with HIV means that policy makers do not need to consider persistent HIV stigma and legal risk, which is evident by the large number of states that still have criminal laws that punish HIV nondisclosure (Center for HIV Law and Policy, 2018).

This matrix of socio-political issues also informs the usage of and belief that molecular HIV surveillance will work. I have argued that the turn toward a form of 'molecular truth-telling' might risk overriding the individuals' sense of sexual identity, desires and notions of how to balance risk and pleasure if not navigated carefully. Molecular HIV surveillance is indeed a potent form of surveillance, however, its many unintended ethical pitfalls should make us question its usage, as well as insist on a clear ethical and legal framework built upon an engagement with stakeholders as well as research communities in such a fashion that we do not end up with a panoptic molecular form of surveillance, a form of 'truth-telling' which ends up stigmatizing communities.

Notes

1 See the CDC information sheet about this; https://www.cdc.gov/hiv/programresources/guidance/molecular-cluster-identification/qa.html
2 See the CDC Q&A on molecular surveillance; https://www.cdc.gov/hiv/programresources/guidance/molecular-cluster-identification/qa.html
3 See the CDC Q&A on molecular HIV surveillance; https://www.cdc.gov/hiv/programresources/guidance/molecular-cluster-identification/qa.html
4 See the Center for HIV Law and Policy; http://www.hivlawandpolicy.org/sites/default/files/CHLP%20Molecular%20Surveillance%20Final.pdf

References

Armstrong, David (1995). The rise of surveillance medicine, *Sociology of Health and Illness*, *17*(3), 393–404.

Bernard, E. J., Azad, Y., Vandamme, A.-M., Weait, M., & Geretti, A. M. (2007). HIV forensics: Pitfalls and acceptable standards in the use of phylogenetic analysis as evidence in criminal investigations of HIV transmission. *HIV Medicine*, *8*(6), 382–387.

Boulton, M., Hart, G., & Fitzpatrick, R. (1992). The sexual behavior of bisexual men in relation to HIV transmission. *AIDS Care*, *4*(2), 165–175.

Castor, D., Low, A., Evering, T., Karmon, S., Davis, B., Figueroa, A., ... Markowitz, M. (2012). Transmitted drug resistance and phylogenetic relationships among acute and early HIV-1-infected individuals in New York City. *Journal of Acquired Immune Deficiency Syndromes (1999)*, *61*(1), 1–8.

Center for Disease Control (2018). *Detecting and Responding to HIV Transmission Clusters. A Guide for Health Departments*. Washington D.C.: CDC.

Center for HIV Law and Policy. (2018). Is molecular HIV surveillance worth the risk? Retrieved from http://www.hivlawandpolicy.org/sites/default/files/CHLP%20Molecul ar%20Surveillance%20Final.pdf.

Chaillon, A., Essat, A., Frange, P., Smith, D. M., Delaugerre, C., Barin, F. (2017). Spatiotemporal dynamics of HIV-1 transmission in France (1999–2014) and impact of targeted prevention strategies. *Retrovirology*, *14*(1), 15. https://doi:10.1186/s12977-017-0339-4

Chow, E. P., Wilson, D. P., & Zhang, L. (2011). What is the potential for bisexual men in China to act as a bridge of HIV transmission to the female population? Behavioural evidence from a systematic review and meta-analysis. *BMC Infectious Diseases*, *11*, 242.

Coltart, C. E., Hoppe, A., Parker, M., Dawson, L., Amon, J. J., Simwinga, M., ... & Eba, P. (2018). Ethical considerations in global HIV phylogenetic research. *The Lancet HIV*, *5*(11), e656–e666.

Da Silva, Chantal. (2018). Donald Trump says immigrants bring 'large scale crime and disease' to America in *Newsweek*. Retrieved from https://www.newsweek.com/donald-trump-says-migrants-bring-large-scale-crime-and-disease-america-1253268.

Dean, T. (2015). Mediated intimacies: Raw sex, Truvada, and the biopolitics of chemoprophylaxis. *Sexualities*, *18*(1–2), 224–246.

Dennis, A. M., Hué, S., Pasquale, D., Napravnik, S., Sebastian, J., Miller, W. C., & Eron, J. J. (2015). HIV transmission patterns among immigrant Latinos illuminated by the integration of phylogenetic and migration data. *AIDS Research and Human Retroviruses*, *31*(10), 973–980.

Epstein, S. (1996). *Impure science: AIDS, activism, and the politics of knowledge*. Berkeley, CA: University of California Press.

Farmer, P. (2006). *AIDS and accusation: Haiti and the geography of blame*. Berkeley, CA: University of California Press.

Foucault, M. (2002). *The birth of the clinic*. London: Routledge.

Gagnon, M., & Guta, A. (2012a). Mapping community viral load and social boundaries: geographies of stigma and exclusion. *Aids*, *26*(12), 1577–1578.

Gagnon, M., & Guta, A. (2012b). Mapping HIV community viral load: space, power and the government of bodies. *Critical Public Health*, *22*(4), 471–483.

German, D., Grabowski, M. K., & Beyrer, C. (2017). Enhanced use of phylogenetic data to inform public health approaches to HIV among men who have sex with men. *Sexual Health*, *14*(1), 89–96.

González-Alba, J. M., Holguín, A., Garcia, R., García-Bujalance, S., Alonso, R., Suárez, A., ... García-Bermejo, I. (2011). Molecular surveillance of HIV-1 in Madrid, Spain: A phylogeographic analysis. *Journal of Virology*, *85*(20), 10755–10763.

González-Alba, J. M., Holguín, A., Garcia, R., García-Bujalance, S., Alonso, R., Suárez, A., . . . García-Bermejo, I. (2011). Molecular surveillance of HIV-1 in Madrid, Spain: A phylogeographic analysis. *Journal of Virology*, *85*(20), 10755–10763.

Guta, A., Gagnon, M., Mannell, J., & French, M. (2016a). Gendering the HIV "Treatment as prevention" paradigm: Surveillance, viral loads, and risky bodies. In: *Expanding the Gaze Gender and the Politics of Surveillance*, edited by van der Meulen, Emily and Heyen, Robert, 156–184. Toronto: University of Toronto Press.

Guta, A., Murray, S. J., & Gagnon, M. (2016b). HIV, viral suppression and new technologies of surveillance and control. *Body & Society*, *22*(2), 82–107.

Han, C.-S. (2015). No brokeback for black men: Pathologizing black male (homo) sexuality through down low discourse. *Social Identities*, *21*(3), 228–243.

Hué, S., Brown, A. E., Ragonnet-Cronin, M., Lycett, S. J., Dunn, D. T., Fearnhill, E., … Delpech, V. C. (2014). Phylogenetic analyses reveal HIV-1 infections between men misclassified as heterosexual transmissions. *AIDS*, *28*(13), 1967–1975.

Huet, T., Cheynier, R., Meyerhans, A., Roelants, G., & Wain-Hobson, S. (1990). Genetic organization of a chimpanzee lentivirus related to HIV-1. *Nature*, *345*(6273), 356.

Ingram, A. (2008). Domopolitics and disease: HIV/AIDS, immigration, and asylum in the UK. *Environment and Planning D: Society and Space*, *26*(5), 875–894.

Kempner, Martha (2019). New study triggers concerns over use of molecular HIV surveillance in *the BodyPro*. Retrieved from https://www.thebodypro.com/article/concerns-over-use-of-molecular-hiv-surveillance.

Lai, A., Bergna, A., Simonetti, F. R., Franzetti, M., Bozzi, G., Micheli, V. … Ciccozzi, M. (2020). Contribution of transgender sex workers to the complexity of the HIV-1 epidemic in the metropolitan area of Milan. *Sexually Transmitted Infections*. Online First.

Little, S. J., Pond, S. L. K., Anderson, C. M., Young, J. A., Wertheim, J. O., Mehta, S. R., … Smith, D. M. (2014). Using HIV networks to inform real-time prevention interventions. *PloS one*, *9*(6), e98443.

McClelland, A., Guta, A., & Gagnon, M. (2019). The rise of molecular HIV surveillance: implications on consent and criminalization. *Critical Public Health*, 1–7.

Mehta, S. R., Schairer, C., & Little, S. (2019). Ethical issues in HIV phylogenetics and molecular epidemiology. *Current Opinion in HIV and AIDS*, *14*(3), 221–226.

Mindock, Clark. (2017). Donald Trump suggested Haitian immigrants to the US 'all have AIDS', officials claim. *The Independent*. Retrieved from https://www.independent.co.uk/news/world/americas/us-politics/donald-trump-suggested-haitian-immigrants-have-aids-officials-claim-a8126861.html.

Montgomery, J. P., Mokotoff, E. D., Gentry, A. C., & Blair, J. M. (2003). The extent of bisexual behaviour in HIV-infected men and implications for transmission to their female sex partners. *AIDS Care*, *15*(6), 829–837.

Novas, C., & Rose, N. (2000). Genetic risk and the birth of the somatic individual. *Economy and Society*, *29*(4), 485–513.

Oster, A. M., France, A. M., & Mermin, J. (2018a). Molecular epidemiology and the transformation of HIV prevention. *Jama*, *319*(16), 1657–1658.

Oster, A. M., France, A. M., Panneer, N., Ocfemia, M. C. B., Campbell, E., Dasgupta, S., … Hernandez, A. L. (2018b). Identifying clusters of recent and rapid HIV transmission through analysis of molecular surveillance data. *JAIDS Journal of Acquired Immune Deficiency Syndromes*, *79*(5), 543–550.

Oster, A. M., Wertheim, J. O., Hernandez, A. L., Ocfemia, M. C. B., Saduvala, N., & Hall, H. I. (2015). Using molecular HIV surveillance data to understand transmission between subpopulations in the United States. *Journal of Acquired Immune Deficiency Syndromes* (1999), *70*(4), 444.

Persson, A., & Newman, C. (2008). Making monsters: Heterosexuality, crime and race in recent Western media coverage of HIV. *Sociology of Health and Illness*, *30*(4), 632–646.

Preciado, P. B. (2013). *Testo junkie: Sex, drugs, and biopolitics in the pharmacopornographic era*. New York, NY: The Feminist Press at CUNY.

Poon, A. F., Gustafson, R., Daly, P., Zerr, L., Demlow, S. E., Wong, J., . . . Moore, D. (2016). Near real-time monitoring of HIV transmission hotspots from routine HIV genotyping: An implementation case study. *The Lancet HIV*, *3*(5), e231–e238.

Rabinow, P., & Rose, N. (2003). *Thoughts on the concept of biopower today*. The Molecular Sciences Institute, 1.

Rabinow, P., & Rose, N. (2006). Biopower today. *BioSocieties, 1*(2), 195–217.

Ragonnet-Cronin, M., Hodcroft, E. B., & Wertheim, J. O. (2019a). Understanding disclosed and cryptic HIV transmission risk via genetic analysis: What are we missing and when does it matter? *Current Opinion in HIV and AIDS, 14*(3), 205–212.

Ragonnet-Cronin, M., Hu, Y. W., Morris, S. R., Sheng, Z., Poortinga, K., & Wertheim, J. O. (2019b). HIV transmission networks among transgender women in los Angeles County, CA, USA: A phylogenetic analysis of surveillance data. *Lancet HIV, 6*(3), e164–e172.

Ragonnet-Cronin, M., Hué, S., Hodcroft, E. B., Tostevin, A., Dunn, D., Fawcett, T. … Brown, A. J. L. (2018). Non-disclosed men who have sex with men in UK HIV transmission networks: Phylogenetic analysis of surveillance data. *Lancet HIV, 5*(6), e309–e316.

Rose, N. (2007). Molecular biopolitics, somatic ethics and the spirit of biocapital. *Social Theory and Health, 5*(1), 3–29.

Sangaramoorthy, T. (2014). *Treating AIDS: Politics of difference, paradox of prevention*. New Brunswick: Rutgers University Press.

Schneider, Jacob, & Birnbaum, Jeffery (2019). The wrong way to 'improve' HIV testing in *the New York Post*. Retrieved from https://nypost.com/2019/05/17/the-wrong-way-to-improve-hiv-testing/.

Snow, J. A. D. T. (1855). *On the mode of communication of cholera, by John Snow, much enlarged* (2nd ed.). London: J. Churchill (London).

Stone, B. E. (2011). The down low and the sexuality of race. *Foucault Studies*, (12), 36–50.

Tani, Maxwell (2015). Paul LePage blames undocumented immigrants for spreading disease in *the Huffington Post*. Retrieved from https://www.huffpost.com/entry/paul-lepage-immigration-disease_n_6616000?guce_referrer=aHR0cHM6Ly93d3cuZ29vZ2xlLmNvbbS8&guce_referrer_sig=AQAAALjf8HZcy54yQo5tknth1EROHyBAkQJuVDJjMpvt44G65zHrxd2QUXvfQdRkuFRvvfEVVDEpPES5rouzjryy1C8A-z4x4Ax_0pzCebzplvifwrjZVk2FYmAIU_e1-2vM_1i4Zo46UkcxDRLAQ-AKSAeQUByE6aGeaGJuofPCJgyS&guccounter=2.

Taylor, B., & Sapién, H. (2020). Determining the direction of HIV transmission: Benefits and potential harms of taking phylogenetic analysis one step further. *Clinical Infectious Diseases*.

Tondo, Lorenzo (2018). Italy orders seizure of migrant rescue ship over 'HIV-contaminated' clothes in *The Guardian*. Retrieved from https://www.theguardian.com/world/2018/nov/20/italy-orders-seizure-aquarius-migrant-rescue-ship-hiv-clothes.

Treichler, P. A. (1999). *How to have theory in an epidemic: Cultural chronicles of AIDS*. Durham: Duke University Press.

Wintour, Patrick (2014). Nigel Farage defends plan to bar immigrants with HIV from NHS care in *The Guardian*. Retrieved from https://www.theguardian.com/politics/2014/oct/10/nigel-farage-defends-plan-immigrants-hiv-nhs.

Wirden, M., De Oliveira, F., Bouvier-Alias, M., Lambert-Niclot, S., Chaix, M.-L., Raymond, S., . . . Bellecave, P. (2019). New HIV-1 circulating recombinant form 94: From phylogenetic detection of a large transmission cluster to prevention in the age of geosocial-networking apps in France, 2013 to 2017. *Eurosurveillance, 24*(39).

Wood, R. W., Krueger, L. E., Pearlman, T. C., & Goldbaum, G. (1993). HIV transmission: Women's risk from bisexual men. *American Journal of Public Health, 83*(12), 1757–1759.

Part III

Targeting the end of AIDS

Genuine solidarity and empowerment or individualized responsibility?

5 PrEP
The public life of an intimate drug

Introduction

Writing a book on the 'end of AIDS' in 2019 and 2020 seems impossible without including a chapter on one of the most visible and debated prevention tools that has emerged in the history of the HIV epidemic. I am here referencing the discovery, development and rollout of pre-exposure prophylaxis (PrEP) for HIV.

In the absence of a cure or a vaccine for HIV, the end of AIDS discourse has relied increasingly on the treatment as prevention (TasP) paradigm as well as the so-called 'test, treat and retain' strategy. Moreover, in 2012, the narrative of a biomedical end to AIDS was radically boosted when the US Food and Drug Administration (FDA) approved the drug Truvada for PrEP usage against HIV. If the HTPN 052 trial in 2011 was named *Science* magazine's breakthrough discovery of the year, then the subsequent approval and trial findings of Truvada as a pre-exposure prophylaxis was soon heralded as both a 'revolution' in HIV science, a 'game-changer' and a 'wonder drug' that would truly be the 'magic bullet' that would end AIDS.

Truvada, consisting of the active drugs emtricitabine and tenofovir, had already in 2004 been approved for usage as a treatment option for PLHIV, but through a series of international randomized controlled trials, it was also approved as a pre-exposure prophylactic (PrEP) drug for people at high-risk for HIV transmissions. Clinical trials showed that Truvada as PrEP reduced risk of HIV infections upwards of 99 percent[1] (Grant et al., 2010; McCormack et al., 2016; Molina et al., 2015) if taken as prescribed. 'Taken as prescribed' in this context includes mainly adhering to two different dosing regimens: either daily PrEP or so-called 'on-demand' or intermittent dosing. On-demand dosing requires PrEP users to take 2 pills 2 to 24 hours before sex, then 1 pill 24 hours after sex and then again 1 pill 24 hours after that.[2] In the wake of these two dosing regimens, several other dosing regimens have also been discovered offering different flexibilities for people who are on PrEP.[3] After its initial approval by the FDA and subsequent recommendation from the US CDC, PrEP has become something of a buzz drug in the HIV discourse. Currently, 44 regulatory authorities have approved PrEP and 2 international and 28 national guidelines have been issued on PrEP usage (Pebody, 2018). To this can be added multiple current pilot projects, demonstration projects and clinical trials that are ongoing across the globe in various nations. Per *PrEP Watch*, an online resource made by AVAC, PrEP is currently being used at different scales and in different forms in 77 countries with between 350,000 and 380,000 people on PrEP in one form or another (PrEP Watch, 2020).

While this number might seem large, UNAIDS has stated that they estimate that approximately 3 million people are at high risk of contracting HIV (UNAIDS, 2018:79). In the US, the figure of PrEP users was around 77,000 people per AIDSVu.[4] Yet the US CDC has stated that the number of people they consider high-risk and in need of HIV preventive interventions, including PrEP, is close to 1.2 million people.[5] Gaps in PrEP access vary globally and nationally, but generally, these gaps have been attributed to cost barriers, differing levels of awareness regarding access to PrEP and infrastructural differences in the promotion of PrEP programs and the number of clinics offering counseling and outreach campaigns. In 2018, AIDS advocacy group, ACT UP, noted that PrEP was still too expensive for many people and that cost barrier, even when PrEP was funded through co-payment schemes, was too high for many of those who needed it most in the US (CDC, 2015).

While PrEP has been endorsed as safe, effective and, in most settings, cost-effective, the HIV preventive technology which is often seen as integral to the end of AIDS, its rollout, scale-up and uptake has been uneven, slow and even controversial.

Here I focus on two issues of the PrEP scale-up and its role in the alleged 'end of AIDS' narrative. First, I give an account of PrEP as controversy, that is, I want to highlight how this intimate drug became a public object subjected to an immense 'mediatization' as Briggs and Hallin might have called it (Briggs, 2005; Briggs & Hallin, 2016). In this analysis I dedicate some space to analyzing what has been called 'the Truvada Wars' (Belluz, 2014), i.e., the controversies that arose in the US and UK. With a drug this effective at preventing HIV and boasting a safety profile that produces very few side effects, one would perhaps be excused for thinking that the scale-up of this drug and its usage would generally be applauded and encouraged in unison. Yet this has been far from the case. I argue that this must be seen in the light of the lingering and ongoing signifying epidemic that has been a theme in this book and which builds on Paula Treichler's work (Treichler, 1999). Once again, my argument is that the end of AIDS, as it is currently being constructed, focuses almost exclusively on metrics and indicators which measure and gauge biomedical technologies and their impact on the epidemic. Yet if this was the sole thing that would end AIDS and ensure an 'HIV-free generation', then controversies such as those surrounding PrEP would not play out through often homophobic and discriminating rhetoric and discourses.

I use PrEP as a controversy as a way of illuminating the signifying practices that inform the discourse around PrEP and, in particular, the stigma of HIV, gay male sexuality and its entanglements with issues of austerity and neoliberalism. In this optic then, the end of AIDS is also entangled with a political economy of neoliberalism, with its subsequent focus on individual responsibility, market choice and rational actor theory. In the end, this chapter highlights the public life of an intimate drug, the controversies that it has produced and the many paradoxical fashions in which the freedom it accords also is bound up with medicalized power. While PrEP's role in ensuring the end of AIDS is yet to be written, what can be said at this historical moment is something of the signifying effects that it has currently produced as well as the public life of an intimate drug.

'Truvada whores and the Truvada wars'

One argument in this book is that the 'end of AIDS' narrative and the making of this slogan can be seen as the construction of an idea that most actors can rally around, yet which might signify different things for different actors. The same can be said about PrEP as it was rolled out after its 2012 FDA approval. Ending AIDS as a global epidemic has gathered diverse actors ranging from HIV activists, private pharmaceutical companies, national health authorities, patients' organizations as well as medical communities and research institutions. This alliance is at times antagonistic and tension-filled, and PrEP as controversy is no exception to this. While PrEP has been embraced by many, it has also created controversies as well as speculations and anticipations. Hopes and fears have been actualized through this drug, and it is to these issues I now turn as part of the current cultural chronicle of what it means to end AIDS.

Kane Race has called attention to PrEP as a form of 'reluctant object' in the semiotic economy and practical infrastructure of gay sexuality (Race, 2016, 2017). Race states that PrEP can be seen as a reluctant object as the uptake of PrEP amongst gay communities in the US, UK and Australia was slower than health authorities initially had hoped and thought would be the case (Race, 2016:16). But more importantly, Race suggests, is that PrEP is seen as a reluctant object 'an object that may well make a tangible difference to people's lives, but whose promise is so threatening or confronting to enduring habits of getting by in this world that it provokes aversion, avoidance – even condemnation and moralism' (Race, 2016:17). Furthermore, PrEP as controversy, as an object that inspires hopes as well as fears that play on liberation but also engender feelings of condemnation can be analyzed as an opportunity to think through

> the affective reaction with which news of PrEP is often greeted: a reaction of aversion – often powerful aversion and repudiation […] It might also help frame HIV prevention as a matter of affective attachments and investments: that is, how people come to attach themselves to particular objects, practices, devices, positions and identities in their attempts to avoid – or otherwise navigate – the possibility of HIV infection.
>
> (Race, 2016:17)

This last insight from Race can, I argue, be extrapolated to the larger narrative of what it means to 'end AIDS'; that is, how we think through the many technologies, drugs and surveillance techniques but also community practices, identities and positions as part of an attempt to navigate the 'end of AIDS'. If PrEP can be seen as a reluctant object in the configuration of the end of AIDS, one of the most vocal attacks on it came from Michael Weinstein, president of the AIDS Healthcare Foundation (AHF). The AHF was founded in 1990 as a non-governmental organization (NGO) and is today the largest provider in the US for HIV/AIDS care per the AHF website (AHF, 2020). The AHF is now also a global actor within the drive to 'end AIDS', currently provides care for 1,388,127 clients worldwide, employs about 6,717 people worldwide[6] and enjoys revenues of over a billion dollars.[7] In 2014, Weinstein went on record calling PrEP a 'party drug' (Chiu, 2014), and in 2015 the AHF launched a commercial penned by Weinstein called 'The War Against Prevention', wherein he publically argued that PrEP would detract funding and attention from condom usage. In the advertisement which ran in various media outlets in Chicago, South Florida, San Francisco/Bay Area, Washington DC, Seattle, Dallas, Brooklyn, Los Angeles and New York, Weinstein asked the question of 'What will become of the condom culture that has been so hard-fought since the beginning of AIDS?' (Weinstein, 2015). Weinstein went on to state that

> AIDS Healthcare Foundation is not against PrEP. Truvada can be the right decision for specific patients who, in consultation with their doctors, decide this is the best choice [...] However, the entire body of scientific data demonstrates that Truvada will not be successful as a mass public health intervention. Yet, this is exactly what PrEP advocates, including the Centers for Disease Control and Prevention, recommend.
>
> (Weinstein, 2015)

Weinstein's statements were met with criticism from both medical and gay communities alike; Mark Joseph Stern, writing for Slate.com called Weinstein *the enfant terrible* of AIDS activism and noted that

> Weinstein has taken it upon himself to take the contrarian position, even if that requires mangling and misreporting science. There's an easy solution to this problem: stop reporting Weinstein's nonsense as though it's real commentary. There are, to be sure, some nuanced concerns about Truvada – but its efficacy is no longer one of them. We shouldn't give Weinstein the pleasure of creating a debate where one simply doesn't exist.
>
> (Stern, 2014)

In *Plus Magazine*, an article was written stating that Weinstein's comments were 'anti-scientific', 'sex-negative', 'shaming' and 'fueled by internalized homophobia' (Staley et al., 2015).

However, Weinstein was not alone in criticizing the approval and rollout of PrEP; Richard Weinmeyer, a research associate with the American Medical Association's Ethics Group, published an online article at the *Hastings Center* website called 'Truvada: No Substitute for Responsible Sex' (Weinmeyer, 2014). In this article, Weinmeyer stated that while the scientific evidence that Truvada worked exists, what was lacking was 'a frank discussion about personal responsibility in gay men's sexual health choices and the duties all of us have, not only to ourselves but also to our partners and the gay community as a whole' (Weinmeyer, 2014). Weinmeyer went on to claim that

> The debate about Truvada has not necessarily focused on those who need the drug, however. Instead, it has centered on those who want the drug, specifically, those who want to use Truvada because their condom use is sporadic or simply because they refuse to use condoms at all. For younger men, infrequent condom use may stem from the realization that HIV is no longer the lethal attacker it once was. Whatever the justification is for ditching safer sex practices, the recent evidence of this unhealthy activity is startling and cause for concern, particularly in light of how many men continue to be unaware of their HIV status.
>
> (Weinmeyer, 2014)

Invoking personal responsibility, Weinmeyer seems to play on tropes that divide gay communities into those who 'really need' Truvada (and thus deserve Truvada) and those who 'just want' Truvada, since they sporadically use condoms or even flat-out refuse to use them. In any case, Weinmeyer creates two subject positions, those who are responsible and those who are not. This resonates with the well-known dichotomy between the deserving versus the undeserving poor (Katz, 1989). It also connects to insights from a long strand in HIV social scientific research on how the HIV epidemic has created semiotic dichotomies such as positive/negative, 'clean/dirty', responsible/irresponsible, rational/irrational, moral/immoral and adherent/non-adherent (Cormier McSwiggin, 2017; Kenworthy, Thomann, & Parker, 2018; Sontag, 1989; Treichler, 1999). Weinstein's comment that Truvada is a 'party drug' and Weinmeyer's statement that some gay men only want Truvada as a way of ditching the condom seem to play on the notion of the irresponsible and hedonistic gay man who, with reckless abandon, leaves all notions of responsibility by the wayside. Yet it is interesting that both Weinstein and Weinmeyer create an opposition between, on the one hand, Truvada and, on the other hand, sexual responsibility. Weinmeyer goes in a sense much further than Weinstein in arguing for such a polar opposition between Truvada and sexual responsibility. Weinmeyer writes that 'If some gay men have decided to not use condoms because they no longer fear exposure to HIV, there is a valid concern that this "condom use nonchalance" within the gay community will apply to Truvada use as well' (Weinmeyer, 2014). Weinmeyer seems here to invert an argument used *for* Truvada, namely that Truvada might be a good preventive alternative for those who do not use condoms for some reason or other (Grant & Koester, 2016). However, Weinmeyer's argument only focuses on an alleged group of gay men who have made an *explicit* decision to *not use condoms* since they no longer seem to fear HIV. Hence, his reversal is that if some gay men do not use condoms why would they then want to adhere to regular PrEP regimens?

My analytical departure here is not so much issues of adherence to PrEP, a topic that has garnered both populist attention as well as serious medical attention (Amico & Stirratt, 2014; Golub, Gamarel, Rendina, Surace, & Lelutiu-Weinberger, 2013; Haberer, 2016a). Nor is my interest so much 'condom fatigue' or even 'AIDS optimism' within gay communities (Adam, Husbands, Murray, & Maxwell, 2005; Singer, 1999). Rather, my departure point is to think through the controversies that can be said to lie within Weinstein and Weinmeyer's rhetorical positions in an age wherein the end of AIDS is the common goal. Without psychologizing Weinstein and Weinmeyer in the manner in which *Plus* magazine called out Weinstein as being motivated by 'internalized homophobia', I instead want to disentangle the statements of these two actors and link them to the broader social canvas onto which these echo against.

Weinstein and Weinmeyer argue from two sides of the same coin, I claim; on the one side, Weinstein seems to argue that PrEP as a preventive technology threatens to undermine 'condom culture' as it has emerged in gay communities. Condom culture, that is, the use of condoms during sex within gay communities has for some time been analyzed as one of several sites wherein norms for sexual citizenship and acceptance have been fought within the gay communities (Davis, 2008; Escoffier, 1998; Richardson, 2000). Arguing that the 1960s and 1970s signified the 'sexual revolution' highlighted by the birth control pill, the Stonewall riots and the earlier Compton's Cafeteria riot in San Francisco, these events in sexual and, in particular, LGBTQI culture, opened up what Jeffrey Escoffier argues, was a 'golden age of sexual freedom' (Escoffier, 2011). Escoffier states that it 'was an era that not only opened up the possibility of openly acknowledging one's homosexuality and fostering a sense of identity and community, it also initiated a period of radical sexual experimentation' (Escoffier, 2011:129). Yet the AIDS epidemic, as Escoffier underscores, 'destroyed that Utopian dream' (Escoffier, 2011:129). While I do not think that Escoffier's utopian melancholia is necessarily the only perspective on the configurations that followed in the wake of the HIV/AIDS epidemic, I do think the push for 'safe sex' and subsequent adaptation of sex with condoms is important to think about in trying to understand PrEP as both a controversy and a reluctant object. The notion that PrEP somehow equates to being 'anti-condom' is also seen across different online forums. In an article on the *AIDSMap* web page, we can read echoes of that early controversy and fear that PrEP usage would undermine the condom culture that Weinstein so laments. The article, entitled *PrEP Wars: Debating Pre-exposure Prophylaxis in the Gay Community*, highlights this through a survey of statements taken from gay blogs such as *Towleroad* and *Joe.My.God* (Cairns, 2013). Safe sex in many of these blogs' initial posts was squarely linked to condom usage as can be discerned by the two following statements: 'Condoms are never in the way. That should be the philosophy and the driving force behind all HIV prevention efforts' and '[...] "in the way" just encourages people to think, "Hey, if I find condoms inconvenient, I'll just take this pill..." This leads down the wrong path'(Cairns, 2013). In these statements, condom culture indicates responsibility, and PrEP, it seems, is seen as a threat to this form of prevention. Much like Weinstein's attack on PrEP as a 'party drug', one which he thinks eventually will undermine safe sex, these statements show the initial backlash that arose when PrEP was rolled out.

Of interest, of course, is that such controversies and subsequent reluctance to embrace PrEP came not only from traditional conservatives, which one might expect, but also from some members of the community. Yet my interest is less in the scientific claims here about 'risk compensation', that is, that PrEP would lead to a reduction in condom usage. While some studies have found that some men do engage in some level of risk compensation (Calabrese et al., 2017; Hojilla et al., 2016; Newcomb, Moran, Feinstein, Forscher, & Mustanski, 2018), others have argued that most gay men on PrEP do not (Koester et al., 2017; Marcus et al., 2013). Barring this discussion, my line of thinking of PrEP as a reluctant object and as the controversy is more aimed at drawing out the semiotic meaning-making that goes into this controversy and informs *why* PrEP is such a reluctant object.

Framing the Truvada whore

So far, it is interesting to note the following aspects of what would come to be known as the 'Truvada wars': (i) the fear and lamenting of the displacement of 'condom culture' and the condom as a signifier of sexual responsibility, (ii) the clear indication that PrEP users are gay men who engage in risky sex and, as such, only *want* PrEP but might not *need* it as they could or even *should* use condoms instead; (iii) the construction of a *division* between PrEP and responsibility. PrEP seems almost paradoxically to be framed as a preventive technology that, if used, signifies not responsibility but indeed irresponsibility. This paradoxical construction of PrEP also led to the creation of the slogan 'Truvada whore' that spawned the moniker of the 'Truvada wars'.

The term 'Truvada whore' came to the fore in a piece written in the *Huffington Post* by David Duran called 'Truvada Whores?' (Duran, 2012). In the article, Duran states that

> In my experience, it seems that a good number of those running to get the prescription are gay men who prefer to engage in unsafe practices. [...] So instead of educating and promoting safe sex practices, the FDA is encouraging the continuation of unsafe sex and most likely contributing to the spread of other sexually transmitted infections.
>
> (Duran, 2012)

While this was before all the large RCTs of Truvada's efficacy had finished up, Truvada in 2012 was still known in the medical community to be highly effective. Indeed, Robert Grant, lead investigator of the iPREX study, had already established in the study that risk reduction numbers were in the very high 90 percent range amongst study participants who had active drug levels in their blood (Grant et al., 2010). However, my argument here is not so much the focus on Truvada's efficacy; rather, it is on the semiotic economy it is part of and the effect it has generated as a highlighted public drug.

In the 'Truvada Whores?' article, Durant goes on to note that PrEP usage amongst monogamous gay men, or for sex workers and drug users, is something which represents a clear rational way of using PrEP. However, 'for men who engage in unsafe sex with other men, this is just an excuse to continue to be irresponsible' (Duran, 2012). Finally, this equation with PrEP usage and being irresponsible comes clearly to the fore when Duran states that

> having unprotected sex and willingly taking that risk because you're on an easy, preemptive treatment regime is just plain stupid [...] for gay men who just like bareback sex, Truvada is just an excuse to do what they want to do.
>
> (Duran, 2012)

Much like Weinstein and Weinmeyer, Duran seems to engage in a paradoxical reversal wherein PrEP usage is equated with being irresponsible, while the CDC, much of the medical community and parts of the gay communities in 2012 were heralding PrEP as *the* responsible thing to take to help 'end AIDS'. The entanglement of Truvada and responsibility is a trope that would follow PrEP from its approval in 2012 up until today; in the frame of the 'Truvada whore' discourse, PrEP was framed as both undermining long-standing condom usage and a signifier of respective sexual citizenship. Moreover, it was also framed as fostering a behavior that would lead to an increase in other STIs and HIV incidences if adherence was not optimal. As we shall see later, the notion of responsibility was later also shifted onto ideas of austerity, fiscal responsibility (who should pay for PrEP?) and, in turn, the tension between allocating health resources in an already scarce environment (Hildebrandt, Bode, & Ng, 2019; Lovelock, 2018). This became particularly visible in England and Norway (Sandset, 2019; Sandset & Wieringa, 2019). In fairness to Duran, and as an added analytical point, he did write an opinion piece in the *Huffington Post* in 2014 called *An Evolved Opinion on Truvada*. In the piece, Duran states that through the 'Truvada wars' and in the aftermath of his 'Truvada Whore?' article, his position on Truvada and PrEP has evolved. He states that 'at this point, I am a supporter of anything that will help eliminate future infections'. While it is perhaps interesting in and of itself that Duran changed his position on Truvada over the course of the years, and in line with a steady increase in the effectiveness of PrEP, it is also worth noting that Duran's notion of 'evolved' opinion is also important. Duran's change of mind can perhaps also be read as a way of following how controversies evolve and become entangled with both the ongoing production of evidence and changes in social discourse over time.

Pivoting back to the framing of PrEP as a 'party drug', this also frames PrEP users as gay men who 'do what they want' and that is an 'an easy, preemptive treatment regime'. PrEP users or 'Truvada whores', as the article is titled, are not only shunned and shamed for taking Truvada as a way of engaging in high-risk 'bareback sex', but also framed as people who seem to be 'taking the easy way out'. This was particularly evident in Larry Kramer's words when he stated in the *New York Times*,

> Anybody who voluntarily takes an antiviral every day has got to have rocks in their heads. There's something to me cowardly about taking Truvada

instead of using a condom. You're taking a drug that is poison to you, and it
has lessened your energy to fight, to get involved, to do anything.

(cited in Braun, 2015)

Kramer's statement is perhaps even more virulent than Weinstein's puritan language. Kramer's attack on PrEP also exposes an underlying notion that people
who use PrEP are taking the easy way out and that using PrEP is somehow a form
of capitulating in the fight *against* HIV. In a paradoxical and polemical reversal,
Kramer seems to posit a drug that *prevents* HIV as an object that will undermine
the 'battle' or the effort to end AIDS. Ending AIDS through PrEP it seems, is a
normative and moral issue.

However, it is worth noting that for Kramer this might also be connected to
his long-standing mistrust with the pharmaceutical industry. Kramer started his
career with ACT UP in New York where he, alongside other ACT UP activists, claimed that even LGBTQI-friendly pharmaceutical companies were not
automatically a guarantee to access to lifesaving drugs for PLHIV and that the
market-friendly mechanisms of patents and drug prices meant that disparities
in health care further perpetuated the HIV epidemic (France, 2016). In light of
this, Kramer's statements might be read in a slightly different light, yet its out-
right condemnation of PrEP users as people who seem to be both lazy and not
doing anything should be inserted into the broader semiotic economy of which
PrEP is a part.

Furthermore, in many of the outtakes in the above, PrEP users also seem to be
framed as people who no longer fear HIV, people who have forgotten or never
experienced the dread and fear of HIV. It seems that this too factors into the construction of the Truvada whore; someone who no longer fears HIV, someone who,
as Duran states, has adopted a 'there's a pill for that attitude' (Duran, 2012). Both
Duran and Weinmeyer state that they are glad that HIV is no longer the death
sentence it once was and that stigmas are declining, yet both seem to construct
PrEP users as people who have taken this too far. I argue that at the same time
Duran and Weinmeyer construct HIV as a disease that is still exceptional, they
acknowledge the historical development that ARV treatment has given PLHIV.
Yet in so doing, PrEP users become the 'unworthy', people who have forgotten
the condom, the historical legacy of HIV and their responsibility. It is in this
matrix that the 'Truvada whore' emerges.

Reclaiming the inner whore in the name of prevention

Not long after the above-mentioned public discourse around 'Truvada whores',
the hastag #TruvadaWhore emerged on Twitter. This signaled a process of
reclaiming what Spideldenner has called 'the inner whore' (Spieldenner,
2016:1692). The moniker 'Truvada whore' is a form of 'slut-shaming'. Slut-
shaming is, in feminist literature, a form of controlling and reconfiguring female
sexual liberation through recourse to the figure of the slut (Dow & Wood, 2014;
Ringrose & Renold, 2012). As Ringrose and Renhold state, the figure of the

slut as portrayed as a woman is a figure who cannot be trusted and must be shunned (Ringrose & Renold, 2012). In the above, the Truvada whore is framed as someone who takes 'preemptive shortcuts' to safe sex, has forgotten or takes lightly both HIV and perhaps even the historical legacy of HIV, is risk willing and thus irresponsible. The perhaps ironic reversal is that a prophylactic drug against HIV suddenly becomes associated with being 'slutty', or a 'whore'. Moreover, it is interesting to note, as Spieldenner does, that this construction of PrEP users as slutty and irresponsible has in the past also been accorded to people living with HIV (Spieldenner, 2016:1691). This has also been noted by other scholars who highlight the social construction of people living with HIV as irresponsible, hedonistic and promiscuous (Epstein, 1996; Treichler, 1999). In this semiotic economy, the signifying function of PrEP suddenly emerges alongside older tropes in the HIV epidemic of PLHIV as being promiscuous and irresponsible. This is a rather paradoxical manner of connecting a prophylactic drug meant to prevent HIV to tropes utilized to often demonize and shame people living with HIV.

Returning to the reclaiming of #TruvadaWhore, Calabrese and Underhill have made a call to 'destigmatize Truvada whores' (Calabrese & Underhill, 2015). In their analysis, part of the process of destigmatizing PrEP usage might go through what they call 'prevention identity' (Calabrese & Underhill, 2015:1960). In this optic, PrEP usage, through the reclaiming of the moniker 'Truvada whore' might go through the same process that condom usage did in the earlier days of the HIV epidemic. Indeed, after the emergence of the hashtag #TruvadaWhore on Twitter, we can see traces of this reclaiming and destigmatization across the Internet. Case in point is the light blue t-shirts that emerged with '#TruvadaWhore' across the chest,[8] The t-shirt has become emblematic of reclaiming the moniker of 'Truvada whore' as a form of 'prevention identity'. The t-shirt was launched by Adam Zeboski who, in 2014, started selling the t-shirt (Parsley, 2014). Zeboski stated in an interview that part of his motivation for launching the t-shirt was 'to take that term and transform it and reclaim it as the gay community has done with queer and dyke. Now people are using it as a term of endearment' (Parsley, 2014). With direct reference to the historical reclamation of queer and dyke, Zeboski inscribes 'Truvada whore' into the tradition of re-appropriating and reclaiming terms whose origins were at first derogatory (Rand, 2014). The controversial position of PrEP in this context shows how PrEP and its signifying economy intersects with several domains at once. It intersects with the biomedical framing of it through how effective it is, yet this is far from the whole story as we have seen in the above. PrEP as a speculative object also informs how it was received and how it came to be such a controversial and reluctant object of discourse within the narrative of ending AIDS.

Even the end of AIDS seems to be subject to a normative discourse, that is, even the end of AIDS seems to instill ideas of *how, who and in which ways* AIDS is to be ended. Michael Lucas, another PrEP activist, stated in an article with the *South Florida Gay News*

I do this because I care about the community and I want other people to use PrEP as well. Because I know that if every gay man is taking PrEP there will be no HIV. It will be the end of HIV.

(Parsley, 2014)

Linking PrEP to the end of AIDS, Lucas seems to indicate that PrEP signifies the end of AIDS. If we juxtapose this with the rhetoric fielded by Weinstein, Weinmeyer and others, we see the different positions on PrEP, but, more so, we see the different ways in which PrEP is enacted. In the frame exposed by Weinstein and others, PrEP signifies a loss of responsibility, of progress gained in both instilling normative safe sex practices but perhaps also a loss of historical remembrance of the HIV epidemic as well as a loss of fear of HIV. Conversely, in the frame of reference that is used by, for example, Lucas and Zeboski, PrEP is an object that represents progress: progress toward the end of AIDS, progress in lifting fear that is associated with having sex and progress toward a new form of liberation.

In the tension between Weinstein, Weinmeyer and Kramer on the one hand, and Lucas and Zeboski on the other hand, there is an interesting battle over not only the public health impact of PrEP but indeed, a battle over what PrEP can and should signify, in particular for gay communities. For Kramer and Weinstein, it seems to trigger a form of nostalgia for HIV activism in the 1980s and early 1990s. In this frame of reference, PrEP signifies the easy way out, surrendering to biomedicine and the disengagement with the history and activism of HIV. The loss of condom culture can in this instance be seen as a form of nostalgia triggered by the perceived loss of an important affectual object within gay sexual cultures – the condom. As Lachenal and Mbodj-Pouye write in a slightly different setting, nostalgia should be seen as a complex political effect which brings together 'active practice of regret' with stakes of 'belonging and community' and the 'materiality of nostalgic attachments' (Lachenal & Mbodj-Pouye, 2014). The introduction of PrEP, in the eyes of some, seems to trigger a fear of the condom culture instilled as a response to the HIV epidemic; and the affective responses to PrEP can, I argue, clearly be seen in the responses levied by Weinstein, Weinmeyer and Kramer. Through the nostalgic connection to condom culture, proponents who fear that PrEP will undermine condom usage not only seem to fear the increase in other STIs but also seem to lament the condom as a signifier of responsibility, safety and perhaps even a link to the activism of an earlier age in the HIV epidemic. Larry Kramer's statement that taking PrEP is proof that PrEP 'has lessened your energy to fight, to get involved, to do anything' seems also to bespeak of a fear that HIV activism will be undermined and made, perhaps, undetectable through what he sees as 'the easy way out'. In a slightly different setting, Gabriel Girard has argued that in the age of ending AIDS, an age that focuses almost entirely on biomedical solutions to the problem of HIV, there has been an 'increasing erasure of contemporary experiences of the sickness [HIV/AIDS]. At a time when we have the means to render HIV biologically undetectable, I propose to explore another of the virus's materialities: its social and historic inscription in urban settings' (Girard, 2016:72). Girard's ethnography focuses mainly on how HIV in gay communities in Montreal is inscribed, becomes visible and invisible in various settings in the city. In the age of ending AIDS through biomedical interventions and technological innovations, Girard argues that there is an ongoing erasure of the visible signs of the HIV epidemic. In a way, this might remind us of Kramer's fear and lamentation of PrEP as a drug that threatens to pacify, lessen the will to fight and thus undermine HIV activism. PrEP in this analytic can be seen as an object that ultimately will undermine HIV activism and render invisible and erase the traces of condom culture, HIV activism and the history of the epidemic.

For Lucas and Zeboski on the other hand, PrEP signifies progress, vitality and engagement. As Zeboski stated in an interview, PrEP and the discourse around 'Truvada Whore?', 'inspired me to start the campaign and I'm very excited about the future of PrEP and what it means for HIV prevention and the inevitable end of HIV/AIDS' (Duran, 2014). For Lucas and Zeboski, PrEP signifies not the death or erasure of HIV activism, rather it is an instance of reinvigorated HIV activism and outreach work. Where Kramer and others fear the end of activism and the erasure of condom culture, Zeboski sees it as a form of a progressive treatment regime that not only has the potential to end AIDS but indeed as a source of inspiration. Diametrically opposing views on not only the biomedical properties of PrEP but also what it signifies bespeaks a form of duality in the controversy surrounding PrEP. For some, it is a threat to longstanding and hard-fought recognitions. For others, it represents freedom, progress and a new form of vitality. In some ways, PrEP acts as a form of *pharmakon*: a cure, a poison and a scapegoat.

PrEP: poison, cure and the scapegoating of PrEP users

Pharmakon (derived from Greek) is a composite word that means cure, poison and scapegoat. In the first two meanings of the word, its meaning is taken from everyday pharmacology wherein a drug can be *both* a cure and a poison. An example of this, described by Asha Persson, is how in certain cases ARVs produce HIV-associated lipodystrophy wherein there is a loss of fat in the face, buttocks and arms (Persson, 2004). For Persson, ARVs are *both* cure and poison, but that

> the ambivalent quality of *pharmakon* is more than purely a matter of 'wrong drug, wrong dose, wrong route of administration, wrong patient'. Drugs, as is the case with antiretroviral therapy, have the capacity to be *beneficial and detrimental to the same person at the same time.*
>
> (Persson, 2004:49)

In much the same way, PrEP as a signifying object seems to be both a cure and a poison, both dangerous and liberating depending on the context of the discourse. This is also seen in biomedical terms when debates emerge on whether PrEP will lead to *increases* in other STIs as it *reduces* HIV incidences.

The third meaning of the word *pharmakon* is also useful for us here, namely scapegoating. In this sense, as Boucher and Roussel note, the 'pharmakon was usually a symbolic scapegoat invested with the sum of the corruption of a community. Seen as a poison, it was subsequently excluded from a community in times of crisis as a form of social catharsis, thus becoming a remedy for the city' (Boucher & Roussel, 2007:130). In perhaps a too philosophical analysis of PrEP, I want to argue that in the framework of Kramer and Weinstein, PrEP users are made into scapegoats who are framed as responsible for the decline in condom culture, surrender of HIV activism, alleged increases in other STIs and the decline in morality, as Weinmeyer stated. Kane Race might have called PrEP a 'reluctant object' and to a certain degree this is true, but PrEP I argue has also become a reluctant object through how it has been framed as a cure, a poison and a scapegoat through the labeling of PrEP users as 'Truvada whores'. PrEP as pharmakon is illustrative as it highlights how one and the same drug can have multiple signifying meanings at once. While I don't want to force the analytical point of PrEP as pharmakon I do think its function as a form of scapegoat is highly telling; by pundits such as Kramet and Weinstein, PrEP users became the scapegoats of falling morals, reduced activism and indeed loss of respectability, literally turning, in Duran's phrase, into whores. However, conversely, pro-PrEP users also rely on scapegoating.

Lucas ends his interview with an interesting quote when he states that 'Today a gay man that has no idea about PrEP is scandalous [...] It's [is] preposterous' (Parsley, 2014). While this is anecdotal, we might speculate that new forms of normative prevention identities and communities might emerge as PrEP is rolled out. Lucas' statement that a gay man who has no idea about PrEP as being scandalous or preposterous might reverse PrEP *users as scapegoats*. More research is needed on the topic, but it might be worth investigating how PrEP non-users are being perceived and meet by PrEP users. Will PrEP non-users become the outsiders of new prevention communities within gay and transgender communities? Will a new hierarchy be established wherein PrEP becomes the new norm for HIV prevention?

PrEP use in this optic is framed as highly normative prevention technology, indeed, in perhaps an ironic turn of events, the reclamation of 'Truvada whore' as a positive might run the risk of becoming itself a normative injunction for gay men. I am not arguing against PrEP – far from it. Instead, I am interested in the semiotic economy of how PrEP has come to signify so much more than HIV prevention, to highlight how PrEP is inserted into a broader frame of 'sero normativity'. That is, the possibility and indeed emerging discourse that what counts as 'successful' HIV treatment *always* must mean reaching undetectable viral load levels and subsequently, that those who cannot for whatever reasons not reach undetectable levels, become labeled as 'difficult' and 'non-compliant' (Cormier McSwiggin, 2017). If this is the case in the lives of PLHIV, that biosociality is predicated upon the achievement of undetectable viral loads, what then of those gay men and transgender women who for whatever reasons do *not* go on PrEP? Is there a risk that this controversial drug also will, or even has started to, form a normative *preventive* hierarchy? Leaving out this question, it is clear that PrEP comes with a broad range of moral and affective entanglements.

Marx on PrEP?

In an interesting piece published online by the *Pacific Standard*, the author high-lights both PrEP's normativity and its implications for class and racial inequal-ity. Access to and usage of Truvada was in the beginning, and is still, somewhat devoid of perspectives of how this semiotic economy is often blind to the class aspects of PrEP. While there are multiple studies on the cost-effectiveness of PrEP implementation (Drabo, Hay, Vardavas, Wagner, & Sood, 2016; Koppenhaver, Sorensen, Farnham, & Sansom, 2011; Schackman & Eggman, 2012) and a large discussion on who should pay for PrEP in, for instance, England (Sandset & Wieringa, 2019), less has been written about how class intersects with the sig-nifying economy of PrEP. PrEP, due to its cost, often presupposes that its users can afford to pay for PrEP or are covered by insurance that offers PrEP. This is particularly true in the US.

Since PrEP treatment is often prohibitively expensive, the discourse around use, access, and even the very figure of the Truvada whore must also be under-stood as a question of economy and class. As the *Pacific Standard* article argues, 'Without an emphasis on equal access and democratization of how drugs are developed and produced, the language of AIDS activism can be hijacked by the language of consumer autonomy, which uplifts only some members of the LGBTQ community'(Braun, 2015). In a harsh critique of the economic inequali-ties and access issues connected to PrEP, the author also highlights an important aspect of the very possibility of becoming a PrEP user. Sexual autonomy medi-ated by the access and use of PrEP is at the heart of PrEP discourses. PrEP use is seen as being a rational thing to do in as much as it keeps the subject safe from HIV transmission as well as overall sexual health and wellbeing. Furthermore, it highlights sexual autonomy by framing PrEP use as taking control over one's own sexual health. Yet, this cannot be divorced from issues of consumer economy: without consumer autonomy, sexual autonomy seems less feasible. PrEP as part of the marketplace of prevention clearly links sexual autonomy with economic capacity and thus consumer autonomy.

It is worth having this in mind when we think through why PrEP has become such a public controversy as well as a reluctant object: for many, the controversy is not about the decision to go on PrEP or not, to be a Truvada whore or not. Nor is the object of PrEP as reluctant object due to the many semiotic and signifying aspects that are attached to it. No, the controversy is that far too few actually can access it due to economic disparities and access to health care.

The reluctance to go on PrEP might indeed stem, for some, from an acknowl-edgment that one might not have insurance the next month or be able to afford the follow-up visits with the doctor. It might be that co-payments for PrEP treatment might be too large for the person to carry. As such, any analysis of the discourse of 'Truvada whore' should also come to terms with the very notion of being *able* to *choose* to reclaim that identity and that slogan. For many, this is simply not possible within some health care systems in the world and, in particular, in the US. As Aaron Braun, the author of the *Pacific Standard* article states concerning the early days of ARV treatment access: 'It was clear that there were some who were primarily concerned with consumer autonomy which only made sense for those with means, who could most likely afford the next pharmaceutical cure [...]' (Braun, 2015). The same is also true for PrEP: consumer choice and neoliberal notions of marker options when it comes to HIV prevention lies at the core of many of these issues. To only speak of what PrEP has come to signify within the current discourse of ending AIDS would belie the many structural and economic issues that continue to perpetuate health inequality and access to PrEP. No wonder then, that cost, access, austerity and responsibility also has become part of the 'PrEP as controversy' debate.

Austerity, cost, access and responsibility: whose responsibility and whose risk is it anyway?

If the initial controversy in the US around PrEP was centering on notions of risk compensation, adherence and whether or not PrEP was a 'party drug' that would only increase the incidences of other STIs, then a bit later in England the controversy would center on moral and ethical issues of financing PrEP. In England, like in the US, PrEP as controversy has meant a semiotic economy of meaning-making that has generated normative notions of responsibility and, in many instances, the medicalization of gay male sexuality. PrEP as controversy in England has followed many of the same lines of tension as in the US. However, since the health care systems are different and PrEP was first approved in the US, PrEP as a reluctant object has followed a slightly different trajectory.

As Rusi Jaspal and Birgitte Nerlich have shown in an article on the media coverage of PrEP in the UK when PrEP was rolled out, its reception was divided amongst two lines of framing PrEP (Jaspal & Nerlich, 2017). Broadly speaking, Jaspal and Nerlich state that PrEP in the UK press was framed as either a preventive technology of hope, that is, that PrEP would be a 'revolution', a 'game-changer' and a 'wonder drug' (Jaspal & Nerlich, 2017:484). Another way that PrEP was reported was as a 'weapon against HIV/AIDS' (Jaspal & Nerlich, 2017:486). This metaphor is widespread in the reporting on PrEP and has even found its way into UNICEF blogs where we can read that PrEP is 'a new weapon in the fight against HIV'.[9] Scholarship has long noted the use of military metaphors in the framing of, the immune system made famous by Donna Haraway (Haraway, 1999). It has also been directly linked to how military metaphors have been used and continue to be used as a way of framing global HIV efforts (Nie et al., 2016; Sontag, 2001). It is clear that Paula Treichler's dictum that the HIV epidemic is also an epidemic of signification, and, as such, there is little wonder that metaphors are part of this signifying epidemic. It continues to be so even in our era wherein the end of AIDS is reportedly imminent and that the end of AIDS continues to be thought of and spoken about in terms of 'war', 'fight against HIV' and that we can end AIDS with 'weapons'. Amongst these weapons is, as noted, PrEP.

Yet, amongst the many reports on PrEP as a technology of hope and as a weapon against HIV, Jaspal and Nerlich also found a large body of articles in the popular press that focus on what they call 'risk representations' (Jaspal & Nerlich, 2017:487-488). These reports framed PrEP as a preventive technology that might undermine HIV prevention due to the uncertainty surrounding adherence to the drug and the fear that condoms would be dropped in favor of using only PrEP. Risk compensation also figured heavily in these reports on PrEP, and, as such, we can note many of the same controversies that emerge in the UK and in the US. In terms of how PrEP became a controversy in England, it is worth briefly looking into how the commissioning process of PrEP was conducted and how this became entangled with issues of morals and responsibility.

NHS England versus 'the people': PrEP, policy and uncertainty

While the FDA approved Truvada for PrEP in 2012, the National Health Service England (NHS) waited to see if it could commission PrEP through its system in lieu of the results of the English PROUD study. PROUD was an open-labeled, randomized controlled trial to evaluate PrEP in England through the enrollment of 544 men who have sex with men across 13 sexual health clinics (McCormack et al., 2016). The results of the trial were published when the trial was ended early as analysis showed that PrEP conferred an 86 percent risk reduction in people who took PrEP (McCormack et al., 2016; The Lancet, 2015:e401). Many expected that the NHS would, in light of this, commission PrEP. However, the NHS instead announced on March 21, 2016 that it would not commission PrEP (NHS, 2016). Instead, the NHS stated that it would extend the support and availability of PrEP to the individuals who were part of the PROUD trial and would 'build on the excellent work to date and will be making available up to £2m over the next two years to run several early implementer test sites' (NHS, 2016). Furthermore, the NHS noted that this extension over the next two years would 'seek to answer the remaining questions around how PrEP could be commissioned in the most cost-effective and integrated way to reduce HIV and sexually transmitted infections in those at highest risk' and that this extension would 'aim to test the "real-life" cost-effectiveness and affordability of PrEP as part of an integrated HIV and STI prevention service' (NHS, 2016). In framing the PROUD study in this fashion, the NHS rhetorically stated that there 'were remaining questions around PrEP' about cost-effectiveness and implementation of PrEP in England. In so doing, the NHS England can perhaps be seen as providing us with a rather interesting way of framing the evidence for PrEP's effectiveness. Since the NHS states that it needs more 'local evidence' for the effect of PrEP, the NHS England in a sense seems to indicate that *local particularities* outweigh *notions of universal biomedical evidence*. Uncertainty is here generated by recourse to whether or not PrEP will work in *England and the English context*, not through a universal critique of PrEP's effectiveness in general.

While the NHS acknowledged the evidence generated within the PROUD study, it still maintained that 'longer-term data is needed to be certain that PrEP can make a significant contribution to sexual health and well-being' (NHS, 2016). Furthermore, the statement also noted that it was the responsibility of 'local authorities to be the responsible commissioners for HIV prevention services'

(NHS, 2016). Thus, the NHS moved the responsibility for the funding and the commissioning of PrEP to localized health authorities. The NHS can also be seen to state that while the PROUD study was in line with sound medical evidence generation, it was still not large enough nor was the evidence generated within the study good enough due to the temporal dimension of the trial.

Pivoting back to the NHS' refusal to commission PrEP, the NHS' next framing was to set up a comparison between PrEP and other 'candidate treatments', highlighting that if the NHS were to commission PrEP it might open the door for other treatments currently not on the NHS' commissioning list. This would further strain the NHS's budget leading to hard prioritizations of who should be offered what medical interventions. This, in turn, is not only an explicit statement that there is a danger in commissioning PrEP because it would endanger fiscal budgets but also an explicit statement that certain people with certain illnesses will be impacted by the potential rollout of PrEP.

This soon led to an outcry from medical professionals who argued that PrEP was both effective in real clinical settings and cost-effective vis-a-vis HIV treatment for people who acquire an HIV infection, that PrEP was a preventive tool desired by those who were at risk for an HIV infection and that PrEP had already been implemented in many other countries (McCormack et al., 2016). It also led to a massive call from activists who started groups such as 'PrEPsters' and 'IWantPrEPNow'. This has clear parallels to the formation of various HIV/AIDS activist groups in the 1980s which is perhaps most emblematically represented by the activist group ACT UP. The similarities between the formation of groups such as ACT UP and Project Inform in San Francisco in the 1980s and 1990s and PrEPsters and IWantPrEPNow in England partly overlap in that both ACT UP and PrEPsters work, as Epstein noted in regard to ACT UP, 'to remove bottlenecks in access to HIV treatment, which at first were experimental drugs and later were drugs that had proven efficacy' thus contributing to the notion of 'getting drugs into bodies' (Epstein, 1996:117). This is also what the various PrEP activist groups in England are doing now. By providing online information, using social media and launching campaigns to highlight the benefits of PrEP, who might want to access it and on the other hand, also offering a critical perspective on the NHS rollout of PrEP, PrEP activism follows a long line of groups that have demanded a place at the table. This is done both in terms of policy formation as well as offering a critique of how policy is lagging on the demand of 'getting drugs into bodies'.

However, the NHS, rather than rolling out PrEP through its systems, announced in December 2016 that it would commission a nationwide PrEP trial with 10,000 participants over the next three years to assess how to best implement PrEP within the national context of England and their sexual health clinics.[10] The NHS argued that

> Whilst the efficacy of PrEP has been established in multiple trials across the world, including the PROUD trial that was conducted in England, the relatively small sample prevented the results being generalized to all sexually transmitted infection (STI) clinic attendees and left unanswered key questions about the large-scale use of PrEP. The PrEP Impact Trial aims to

address the outstanding questions about eligibility, uptake, and length of use by expanding the assessment to the scale required to obtain sufficient data.[11]

Furthermore, the NHS argued that the IMPACT trial was important since it would allow 'to answer the key questions under real-world conditions and at a sufficient scale. In addition, the new trial will assess the impact of PrEP on new HIV diagnoses and sexually transmitted infections. The results will inform service commissioners (funders) on how to support clinical and cost-effective PrEP access in the future'.[12]

The announcement was met with what can be seen as a mixed response ranging from the assertion that the IMPACT trial was an important step in the right direction (The Lancet HIV, 2017:e1), to responses demanding that the IMPACT trial consider enrolling other demographic groups outside MSM and transgender women (The Lancet HIV, 2017:e1). The trial has since then been the victim of delays, and enrollment did not start up until October 2017, while it was initially set for enrollments to start in April 2017. Furthermore, the trial was such a success that the original number of people to be included was increased from 10,000 to 13,000 in June of 2018; and, in January 2019, the NHS, once again under pressure from activists' groups, was forced to increase the number of slots within the IMPACT trial from 13,000 to 23,000.[13] However, this extension of the number of slots within the IMPACT trial is so far only provisionally promised, as the NHS notes 'that more work was needed to engage local authority commissioners and ensure that research sites could actually handle the extra capacity'. The lack of slots for participating in the IMPACT trial has led some to observe that people in need of PrEP have been turned away from clinics due to lack of spaces within the trial, thus 'people in need of PrEP will be denied it, and some, as a result, will acquire HIV'.[14]

Responsibility: fiscal and moral?

One of the initial reactions to the NHS decision not to commission PrEP as it is configured in the editorial *PrEP: Why are we waiting?* was to frame the decision within a setting wherein *evidence, efficacy and morality* was entangled as crucial formulation of an evidence-based HIV intervention. The authors framed the inaction of the NHS by referring first to the English PROUD study (McCormack et al. 2016) and its results, which concluded that PrEP was an effective, real-world preventive tool in the fight against HIV (Lancet HIV, 2015:e401). McCormack et al. went on to rally evidence from the US and from the WHO, UNAIDS and AVAC, which they stated had accumulated significant evidence of the real-world effectiveness of PrEP (Lancet HIV, 2015:e401). After this initial recourse to the *amount of evidence as well as the type of evidence*, the authors frame the decision as not only *bad science* but indeed as bad ethics. They stated that

an unmet demand for PrEP and unequal access might lead to people obtaining Truvada through alternative channels without the appropriate counselling or follow-up: by claiming a recent exposure to HIV and receiving the drug for post-exposure prophylaxis from sexual health services or, more damagingly, through an unregulated market that deprives people with HIV of their treatment.

(Lancet, 2015:e401)

Furthermore, this could lead to 'unnecessary delays [which] will lead to HIV infections that could have been prevented' (Jansen et al., 2016:e401). Finally, this example of not listening to 'the growing experience and results from trials and demonstration studies across the world' (Lancet, 2015:e401), would be seen as a failure which 'perpetuates an inequality in access to medicine that will ultimately condemn some people to a lifetime of HIV treatment at enormous expense' (Lancet, 2015:e401). In this line of argumentation, the mixture between evidence and ethics is clear and the authors of the editorial clearly draw on the notion that *enough evidence has been generated* and in fact *experience with PrEP outside RCTs* has also demonstrated this to be effective.

In this editorial, failure to use this evidence is considered immoral and thus ethically dubious. However, in the rebuttal in January of 2016 named *PrEP: Why we are waiting*, (Jansen et al., 2016), morality is framed differently. Here the authors come with a counter claim in terms of morality: *normative social values need to be considered*. In their rebuttal, the authors claim that while *objective evidence* has proven to show the effectiveness of PrEP, *normative aspects* have received little attention, and that such normative aspects as people's own responsibility to use condoms and the relative importance of preventing HIV versus a possible rise in other sexually transmitted diseases because of reduced rates of condom usage must be investigated before one can roll out PrEP (Jansen et al., 2016:e12). The editorial goes on to state that decision-makers do not base their decisions only on the objective aspects of an intervention but are also responsive to normative arguments (Jansen et al., 2016:e12). Before rolling out PrEP, consideration must be given to the 'popular discourse surrounding PrEP' as a 'fun-pill' for people which is taken only by people who want to be promiscuous with little regard for their own responsibility to stay healthy (Jansen et al., 2016:e12). The authors then go on to cite a Dutch study, wherein popular discourse on whether or not PrEP should be publicly reimbursed in the Netherlands was investigated, which they argue confirms that the implementation of PrEP relies on normative aspects of PrEP usage more so than evidence based medicine's claim to effectiveness (Jansen et al., 2016:e12).

No matter the evidence for effectiveness, the authors here invoke morality as a way of postulating that (1) people have a personal responsibility to prevent HIV through condom usage rather than a public health initiative such as PrEP and (2) social norms of morality must be considered in relationship to the implementation of PrEP. Morality is here part of the evidence-making of PrEP; its effectiveness and acceptability are in this frame decided not just by the effectiveness proved within RCTs, but also by normative issues. It is thus immoral *to implement* PrEP without first clarifying *both the objective and the normative* considerations surrounding PrEP (Jansen et al., 2016:e12). The two editorials can be seen as framing evidence and morality in different ways: the editorial whose stand is to roll out PrEP could be taken to argue that it is immoral to *not* implement PrEP *based on* the notion that there indeed *is enough* evidence; and the editorial which argues for the delay of rolling out PrEP might be read as stating that it is a fallacy to *not* consider normative values *as evidence* of a potential implementation of PrEP.

However, social norms were not evoked only within medical editorials. In the popular press, and, in particular, the tabloid press in England, PrEP and the potential commissioning of it through the NHS was picked up as a topic of interest.

In an article published in the Daily Mail, the newspaper described the commissioning of PrEP through the NHS as a strategy that was 'fraught with dangers' such as an upswing in the increase of other STIs, the development of HIV-resistance to drugs due to the scale-up of PrEP and, above all, that the scale-up of PrEP through the NHS would lead to money being taken away from other population groups who were in need of treatments ranging from cancer to cataract treatment (Borland, 2016). The article also cited two spokespersons, one from the Christian Medical Fellowship and another one from the Christian Action Research and Education charity. The spokesperson from the Christian Action Research and Education stated,

> We have really serious concerns about the NHS spending tens of millions on a drug that we believe could facilitate more risky sexual lifestyles. Given the risks of increased promiscuity associated with Prep, this would be an expensive and potentially irresponsible action.
>
> (Borland, 2016)

This was echoed by the spokesperson from the Christian Medical Fellowship who went on to state that

> This is a strategy fraught with dangers. Making PrEP freely available to already promiscuous homosexuals could well encourage more sexual risk taking and more sexually transmitted disease as a result [...] The best way of preventing HIV infections is by avoiding the high-risk sexual behaviours that lead to it. Those who rely on it for protection against HIV are effectively playing Russian roulette.
>
> (Borland, 2016)

In an editorial published in the Telegraph wherein editor Phillipe Johnston proclaimed that

> When the fear of AIDS began in the 1980s everyone was told to change their sexual behaviour even though the people principally at risk were promiscuous homosexuals or intravenous drug users. In order not to moralise about anyone's behaviour we were all required to feel a sense of responsibility.
>
> (Johnston, 2016)

He then went on to connect his refusal to 'shoulder the moral burden' to the NHS commissioning of PrEP by stating that PrEP should not be commissioned because it 'absolves high-risk men from taking precautions like wearing a condom during sex. A spokesman for an AIDS charity said that this was ethically right because we are "all at risk". Really?' (Johnston, 2016).

In these excerpts, the social values held by the spokesperson are entangled with potential clinical outcomes related to PrEP such as an increase in unprotected anal intercourse, an increase in partners and an increase in other STIs. Yet it is also interwoven with the issues of austerity and evaluating which treatments should be given priority. This was echoed by the NHS before the High Court ruled that the NHS was legally allowed to commission PrEP. The NHS stated that rolling out PrEP through the NHS was legally not the responsibility of the nationalized NHS system, rather it was the local commissioning bodies who were responsible for this implementation (NHS, 2016). Furthermore, if the NHS *were* to commission PrEP, this might jeopardize other patient groups who would then have their services competing with PrEP since funding would have to be divided even more than they already were (NHS, 2016). Within the context of the tabloid press, Tory MP Philip Davies was cited as saying that 'There isn't a bottomless pit to spend on the NHS. We've got to prioritise and decide where we should rank this in the list of NHS spending priorities' (Borland, 2016). Clearly, according to the spokespeople from the two Christian organizations, priority within the current austerity climate in the NHS should not be given to PrEP, an issue which was also of concern within the rhetoric of the NHS itself when initially they refused to commission PrEP. In fact, the very article in the Daily Mail was named 'NHS fights back against ruling forcing it to hand out "promiscuity pill" that prevents HIV as the £20m cost will hit its ability to treat cancer and give limbs to amputees'. The very framing of the article clearly casts the commissioning of PrEP as an issue of making a choice between treatments as well as pitting certain population groups against one another – in this case, men who have sex with men versus cancer patients and amputees.

PrEP as controversy in England shows us how evidence, economy and morality become entangled and levied as arguments about PrEP and its commissioning. Moreover, many of the same issues emerged in the case of the US: the notion of PrEP as a 'fun pill', the issue of responsibility and, finally, the moral responsibility to prevent HIV. As such, PrEP as an intimate drug has clearly had a public life that has spawned and re-actualized a broad range of issues, which in turn highlights the tension-filled space that PrEP exists in even in an age that claims to be near the end of AIDS.

Ending AIDS through PrEP: a public controversy over a reluctant object

I have tried in this chapter to map some of the semantic and signifying aspects of the controversies that emerged in the wake of the approval of Truvada as PrEP. In doing so, I sought to draw attention to how the usage of PrEP against HIV in what at first seems like a strange turn of events, elicited an enormous amount of push back. In an era of 'post-AIDS' rhetoric (Ledin & Benjamin, 2019; Persson, Race, & Wakeford, 2003; Race, 2001; Rofes, 2015) combined with a narrative that now increasingly plays on an optimism that we will soon be able to end AIDS, the backlash against PrEP might seem odd. However, as I have tried to show, the stakes of this controversy are multiple and bespeak of the entanglements of older tensions and problems within the HIV epidemic. Old, or perhaps they never left, issues such as the policing of gay sexuality, notions of responsibility between the state and the individual re-emerge in the wake of PrEP. So too did issues concerning autonomy and sexual liberation and its excess. Made anew were issues such as the dichotomies between 'responsible/promiscuous', 'deserving/non-deserving' and 'rational/irrational'.

PrEP as controversy and as a reluctant object of prevention also motivated a new yet familiar debate in HIV science, namely what is considered medical evidence and how to frame this. In the wake of this, issues of fiscal responsibility were also animated yet these responsibilities quickly became moralistic and normative. Tensions regarding the capacities of national health care authorities have been used as rationales for not providing PrEP as we have seen in the case of NHS England. Conversely, activists and the medical community, by and large, have argued that failure to commission PrEP was unethical and irresponsible of the government. The reluctance that Kane Race observed in his scholarship on PrEP (Race, 2016, 2017) is as much about the reluctance to confront sex and sexual pleasure as it is to confront PrEP as such. My analysis has tried to tease this out through different modalities, such as the usage of evidence, the attachment to the condom as a symbol of a normative sexual citizen who is taking responsibility for his and others' sexual health and, finally, how in the end, the reluctance of the NHS to commission PrEP is also a reluctance to spend money in a time wherein austerity has become such a powerful trope that it allows for cuts that in times past would be unthinkable.

The signifying economy that PrEP inserts itself into is thus a re-activated discourse that has been there for a long time within the HIV epidemic. PrEP has allowed for many old entanglements to re-emerge, yet assembled a bit differently, as well as played out in new ways. It represents a controversy that is a controversy not just about HIV prevention, but indeed about gay communities' sexuality and pleasure. If PrEP is one case amongst many that center around the narrative that the end of AIDS is within reach, then PrEP as controversy and as a reluctant object might also tell us something about the larger narrative of ending AIDS. It might tell us that the increased biomedical determinism (i.e., that the end of AIDS will come if only we roll out and scale up HIV testing, ARVs, PrEP and molecular viral surveillance) might be misplaced. Indeed, PrEP as controversy shows us, I argue, that the very notion that the end of AIDS is possible can only be realized if we have politics that acknowledge the HIV epidemic as an epidemic of signification and as an epidemic of materiality. In this realization, a semiotic, post-structural perspective is combined with a Marxist understanding of the economy and the realization that biomedical solutions are key – yet not the only key – to the end of AIDS.

Perhaps PrEP as controversy can shed light on how it has instilled affective responses to gay sexuality, pleasure and intimacy; how it has caused reluctance on the individual and state level (albeit for different yet entangled reasons); and how it has engendered a controversy that sheds light on sexuality and pleasure more broadly. I want to end this chapter by paraphrasing Marx. It might seem like an odd turn, but there is something in Marx' mode of analyzing class struggle and ownership of the means of production which I think can be extrapolated to both PrEP as controversy but also to some general insights for a book concerned with what it can mean to end AIDS.

Marx states in *The German Ideology*,

> The class which has the means of material production at its disposal, has control at the same time over the means of mental production, so that thereby, generally speaking, the ideas of those who lack the means of mental production are subject to it. The ruling ideas are nothing more than the ideal expression of the dominant material relationships, the dominant material relationships grasped as ideas.
>
> (Marx & Engels, 1970)

If we allow ourselves to rethink Marx and Engels here, we might instead state that the class that has the means of material prevention at its disposal has, at the same time, much control over the means of mental production. This has implications for the end of AIDS and PrEP as this also entails that any meaningful discussion about the end of AIDS must take seriously the notion that affected communities must be allowed to co-own the means of *prevention* as well as the means of producing the *narrative* about the end of AIDS. This end to this chapter fuses thus a materialist account of PrEP as controversy with a semiotic account while realizing that co-ownership of both access and use of PrEP is needed as well as co-ownership of the signifying practices that go into narrating both PrEP and the end of AIDS narrative.

Notes

1 See the CDC Fact sheet on PrEP; https://www.cdc.gov/hiv/basics/prep.html
2 See the New York Public Health Department for dosing examples; https://www1.nyc .gov/assets/doh/downloads/pdf/ah/prep-on-demand-dosing-guidance.pdf
3 For a good overview of this, see the iwantprepnow webpage; https://www.iwantpre pnow.co.uk/how-to-take-prep/
4 See the AIDSVu website and subsequent PrEP tracker; https://aidsvu.org/prep/
5 See the CDC's calculation study at the CDC's weekly *Vital Signs*; https://www.cdc .gov/mmwr/preview/mmwrhtml/mm6446a4.htm?s_cid=mm6446a4_w
6 See the AHF webpage for information on these figures and their distribution; https:// www.aidshealth.org/about/
7 See the AHF 2017 revenue forms; https://apps.irs.gov/pub/epostcard/cor/954112121_2 01712_990_2018121916025494.pdf
8 A Google image search yields a host of examples of these t-shirts, for instance, see HIV online magazine; https://www.hivplusmag.com/prevention/2014/06/23/please -feel-free-call-me-truvada-whore

9 See the UNICEF East Asia and Pacific blog spot; https://blogs.unicef.org/east-asia-pacific/preparing-prep-new-weapon-fight-hiv/
10 See the NHS statement on the IMPACT trial and why it is needed; https://www.eng land.nhs.uk/commissioning/spec-services/npc-crg/blood-and-infection-group-f/f03/ prep-impact-trial-questions-and-answers/#what-is-the-prep-impact-trial
11 https://www.england.nhs.uk/commissioning/spec-services/npc-crg/blood-and-infecti on-group-f/f03/prep-impact-trial-questions-and-answers/#what-is-the-prep-impact-trial
12 https://www.england.nhs.uk/commissioning/spec-services/npc-crg/blood-and-infecti on-group-f/f03/prep-impact-trial-questions-and-answers/#what-is-the-prep-impact-trial
13 See the NHS IMPACT updates; https://www.england.nhs.uk/commissioning/spec-serv ices/npc-crg/blood-and-infection-group-f/f03/prep-trial-updates/#june
14 See the NAT's statement on the number of people being turned away due to lack of slots in the IMPACT trial; https://www.nat.org.uk/press-release/first-year-anniversary-openi ng-impact-trial-we-need-end-nhs-rationing-prep

References

Adam, B. D., Husbands, W., Murray, J., & Maxwell, J. (2005). AIDS optimism, condom fatigue, or self-esteem? Explaining unsafe sex among gay and bisexual men. *Journal of Sex Research*, *42*(3), 238–248.

AIDS Healthcare Foundation. (2020). About AHF. Retrieved from https://www.aidshealth .org/about/.

Amico, K. R., & Stirratt, M. J. (2014). Adherence to preexposure prophylaxis: Current, emerging, and anticipated bases of evidence. *Clinical Infectious Diseases*, *59*(suppl_1), S55–S60.

Belluz, J. (2014). The Truvada wars. *BMJ*, *348*, g3811.

Borland, Sophie. (2016). NHS fights back back against rulling forcing it to hand out 'promicuity pill' that prevent HIV as the £20 million cost will hit its ability to treat cancer and give limbs to amputees. *The Daily Mail*. Retrieved from https://www.dai lymail.co.uk/news/article-3720706/What-skewed-sense-values-NHS-told-5-000-year-l ifestyle-drug-prevent-HIV-vital-cataract-surgery-rationed.html.

Boucher, J.-C., & Roussel, S. (2007). From Afghanistan to 'Quebecistan': Quebec as the Pharmakon of Canadian foreign and defence policy. *Canada Among Nations*, 128–142. Norman Paterson School of International Affairs, Carleton University, Montreal.

Braun, Aaron. (2015). 'Truvada Whores' and the class divide. *The Pacific Standard*. Retrieved from https://psmag.com/social-justice/truvada-whores-and-the-aids-class -divide.

Briggs, C. L. (2005). Communicability, racial discourse, and disease. *Annual Review of Anthropology*, *34*(1), 269–291. Retrieved from http://www.jstor.org/stable/25064886

Briggs, C. L., & Hallin, D. C. (2016). *Making health public: How news coverage is remaking media, medicine, and contemporary life*. London: Routledge.

Caims, Gus (2013). PrEP wars: Debating pre-exposure prophylaxis in the gay community in *AIDSMAP*. Retrieved from http://www.aidsmap.com/news/feb-2013/prep-wars-deb ating-pre-exposure-prophylaxis-gay-community.

Calabrese, S. K., Magnus, M., Mayer, K. H., Krakower, D. S., Eldahan, A. I., Hawkins, L. A. G. ... Betancourt, J. R. (2017). 'Support Your Client at the Space That They're in': HIV pre-exposure prophylaxis (PrEP) prescribers' perspectives on PrEP-related risk compensation. *AIDS Patient Care and STDs*, *31*(4), 196–204.

Calabrese, S. K., & Underhill, K. (2015). How stigma surrounding the use of HIV preexposure prophylaxis undermines prevention and pleasure: A call to destigmatize 'Truvada whores'. *American Journal of Public Health, 105*(10), 1960–1964.

Center for Disease Control. (2015). Morbidity and Mortality Weekly Report (MMWR), vital signs: Estimated percentages and numbers of adults with indications for preexposure prophylaxis to prevent HIV acquisition — United States, 2015. Retrieved from https://www.cdc.gov/mmwr/preview/mmwrhtml/mm6446a4.htm?s_cid=mm6446a4_w.

Chiu, Jeff (2014). Divide over HIV prevention drug Truvada persists. *USA Today*. Retrieved from https://eu.usatoday.com/story/news/nation/2014/04/06/gay-men-divided-over-use-of-hiv-prevention-drug/7390879/.

Cormier McSwiggin, C. (2017). Moral adherence: HIV treatment, undetectability, and stigmatized viral loads among Haitians in South Florida. *Medical Anthropology, 36*(8), 1–15.

Davis, M. (2008). The 'loss of community' and other problems for sexual citizenship in recent HIV prevention. *Sociology of Health and Illness, 30*(2), 182–196.

Dow, B. J., & Wood, J. T. (2014). Repeating history and learning from it: What can SlutWalks teach us about feminism? *Women's Studies in Communication, 37*(1), 22–43.

Drabo, E. F., Hay, J. W., Vardavas, R., Wagner, Z. R., & Sood, N. (2016). A cost-effectiveness analysis of preexposure prophylaxis for the prevention of HIV among los Angeles County men who have sex with men. *Clinical Infectious Diseases, 63*(11), 1495–1504.

Duran, David (2012). Truvada whores? *Huffington Post*. Retrieved from https://www.huffpost.com/entry/truvada-whores_b_2113588?guccounter=1.

Duran, David (2014). An evolved opinion on Truvada. *Huffington Post*. Retrieved from https://www.huffpost.com/entry/truvadawhore-an-evolved-o_b_5030285?guce_referrer_us=aHR0cHM6Ly93d3cuZ29vZ2xlLmNvbS8&guce_referrer_cs=i4ShN-aeCgxBLLMoQzrv8A&guccounter=2.

Epstein, S. (1996). *Impure Science: AIDS, activism, and the politics of knowledge* (Vol. 7). Berkeley, CA: University of California Press.

Escoffier, J. (1998). The invention of safer sex: Vernacular knowledge, gay politics and HIV prevention. *Berkeley Journal of Sociology*, Sexuality, *43*, 1–30.

Escoffier, J. (2011). Sex, safety, and the trauma of AIDS. *Women's Studies Quarterly, 39*(1/2), 129–138.

France, D. (2016). *How to survive a plague*. London: Picador.

Girard, G. (2016). *Undetectable? Medicine Anthropology Theory*, 3(3), 72–86.

Golub, S. A., Gamarel, K. E., Rendina, H. J., Surace, A., & Lelutiu-Weinberger, C. L. (2013). From efficacy to effectiveness: Facilitators and barriers to PrEP acceptability and motivations for adherence among MSM and transgender women in New York City. *AIDS Patient Care and STDs, 27*(4), 248–254.

Grant, R. M., & Koester, K. A. (2016). What people want from sex and preexposure prophylaxis. *Current Opinion in HIV and AIDS, 11*(1), 3–9. doi:10.1097/coh.0000000000000216.

Grant, R. M., Lama, J. R., Anderson, P. L., McMahan, V., Liu, A. Y., Vargas, L. … Glidden, D. V. (2010). Preexposure chemoprophylaxis for HIV prevention in men who have sex with men. *New England Journal of Medicine, 363*(27), 2587–2599. doi:10.1056/NEJMoa1011205.

Haberer, J. E. (2016a). Current concepts for PrEP adherence in the PrEP revolution: From clinical trials to routine practice. *Current Opinion in HIV and AIDS, 11*(1), 10–17. doi:10.1097/coh.0000000000000220.

Haberer, J. E. (2016b). Current Concepts for PrEP Adherence: The PrEP revolution; from clinical trials to routine practice. *Current Opinion in HIV and AIDS, 11*(1), 10.

Haraway, D. (1999). The biopolitics of postmodern bodies: Determinations of self in immune system discourse. *Feminist Theory and the Body: A Reader, 1*(1), 203.

Hildebrandt, T., Bode, L., & Ng, J. S. (2019). Responsibilization and sexual stigma under austerity: Surveying public support for government-funded PrEP in England. *Sexuality Research and Social Policy*, 1–11.

Hojilla, J. C., Koester, K. A., Cohen, S. E., Buchbinder, S., Ladzekpo, D., Matheson, T., & Liu, A. Y. (2016). Sexual behavior, risk compensation, and HIV prevention strategies among participants in the San Francisco PrEP demonstration project: A qualitative analysis of counseling notes. *AIDS and Behavior, 20*(7), 1461–1469.

Jaspal, R., & Nerlich, B. (2017). Polarised press reporting about HIV prevention: Social representations of pre-exposure prophylaxis in the UK press. *Health, 21*(5), 478–497.

Johnston, Phillip (2016). We shall not shoulder the moral burden in society's blame game. *The Telegraph*. Retrieved from https://www.telegraph.co.uk/news/2016/08/02/we-shall -not-shoulder-the-moral-burden-in-societys-blame-game/.

Katz, M. B. (1989). *The undeserving poor: From the war on poverty to the war on welfare*, (Vol. 60). New York, NY: Pantheon Books.

Kenworthy, N., Thomann, M., & Parker, R. (2018). From a global crisis to the 'end of AIDS': New epidemics of signification. *Global Public Health, 13*(8), 960–971.

Koester, K., Amico, R. K., Gilmore, H., Liu, A., McMahan, V., Mayer, K. … Grant, R. (2017). Risk, safety and sex among male PrEP users: Time for a new understanding. *Culture, Health and Sexuality, 19*(12), 1301–1313.

Koppenhaver, R. T., Sorensen, S. W., Farnham, P. G., & Sansom, S. L. (2011). The cost-effectiveness of pre-exposure prophylaxis in men who have sex with men in the United States: An epidemic model. *JAIDS: Journal of Acquired Immune Deficiency Syndromes, 58*(2), e51–e52. doi:10.1097/QAI.0b013e31822b74fe.

Lachenal, G., & Mbodj-Pouye, A. (2014). *Politiques de la nostalgie* (Vol. 135). Paris : KARTHALA Editions.

Ledin, C. W., & Benjamin (2019). PrEP at the after/party: The 'post-AIDS' politics of frank ocean's 'PrEP+'. *Somatosphere*. http://somatosphere.net/2019/prep-at-the-after -party.html/

Lovelock, M. (2018). Sex, death, and austerity: Resurgent homophobia in the British tabloid press. *Critical Studies in Media Communication, 35*(3): 1–15.

Marcus, J. L., Glidden, D. V., Mayer, K. H., Liu, A. Y., Buchbinder, S. P., Amico, K. R. … Pilotto, J. (2013). No evidence of sexual risk compensation in the iPrEx trial of daily oral HIV preexposure prophylaxis. *PloS One, 8*(12), e81997.

Marx, K., & Engels, F. (1970). *The German ideology* (Vol. 1). New York, NY: International Publishers Co.

McCormack, S., Dunn, D. T., Desai, M., Dolling, D. I., Gafos, M., Gilson, R. … Gill, O. N. Pre-exposure prophylaxis to prevent the acquisition of HIV-1 infection (PROUD): Effectiveness results from the pilot phase of a pragmatic open-label randomized trial. *Lancet, 387*(10013), 53–60. doi:10.1016/S0140-6736(15)00056-2.

McCormack, S., Dunn, D. T., Desai, M., Dolling, D. I., Gafos, M., Gilson, R. … Schembri, G. (2016). Pre-exposure prophylaxis to prevent the acquisition of HIV-1 infection (PROUD): Effectiveness results from the pilot phase of a pragmatic open-label randomized trial. *Lancet, 387*(10013), 53–60.

Molina, J.-M., Capitant, C., Spire, B., Pialoux, G., Cotte, L., Charreau, I. … Delfraissy, J.-F. (2015). On-demand preexposure prophylaxis in men at high risk for HIV-1 infection. *New England Journal of Medicine, 373*(23), 2237–2246. doi:10.1056/NEJMoa1506273.

National Health Services. (2016). Update on commissioning and provision of Pre Exposure Prophylaxis (PREP) for HIV prevention. Retrieved from https://www.england.nhs.uk /2016/03/prep/.

Newcomb, M. E., Moran, K., Feinstein, B. A., Forscher, E., & Mustanski, B. (2018). Pre-exposure prophylaxis (PrEP) use and condomless anal sex: Evidence of risk compensation in a cohort of young men who have sex with men. *Journal of Acquired Immune Deficiency Syndromes (1999)*, *77*(4), 358–364. doi:10.1097/ QAI.0000000000001604.

Nie, J.-B., Gilbertson, A., de Roubaix, M., Staunton, C., van Niekerk, A., Tucker, J. D., & Rennie, S. (2016). Healing without waging war: Beyond military metaphors in medicine and HIV cure research. *The American Journal of Bioethics*, *16*(10), 3–11.

Parsley, Jason (2014). Truvada whore: The war escalates with AHF's anti-PrEP campaign, *South Florida Gay News*. Retrieved from https://southfloridagaynews.com/National/ truvada-whore-the-war-escalates-with-ahf-s-anti-prep-campaign.html.

Pebody, Roger (2018). 380,000 People on PrEP globally, mostly in the USA and Africa [updated], *AIDSMAP*. Retrieved from https://www.aidsmap.com/news/oct-2018/38 0000-people-prep-globally-mostly-usa-and-africa-updated.

Persson, A. (2004). Incorporating Pharmakon: HIV, medicine, and body shape change. *Body & Society*, *10*(4), 45–67.

Persson, A., Race, K., & Wakeford, E. (2003). HIV health in context: Negotiating medical technology and lived experience. *Health*, *7*(4), 397–415.

PrEP Watch. (2020). *Global Prep Tracker*. Retrieved from https://www.prepwatch.org/ resource/global-prep-tracker/.

Race, K. (2001). The undetectable crisis: Changing technologies of risk. *Sexualities*, *4*(2), 167–189.

Race, K. (2016). Reluctant objects: Sexual pleasure as a problem for HIV biomedical prevention. *GLQ: a Journal of Lesbian and Gay Studies*, *22*(1), 1–31.

Race, K. (2017). *The gay science: Intimate experiments with the problem of HIV*. London: Routledge.

Rand, E. J. (2014). *Reclaiming queer: Activist and academic rhetorics of resistance*. Tuscaloosa, AL: University of Alabama Press.

Richardson, D. (2000). Constructing sexual citizenship: Theorizing sexual rights. *Critical Social Policy*, *20*(1), 105–135.

Ringrose, J., & Renold, E. (2012). Slut-shaming, girl power and 'sexualisation': Thinking through the politics of the international SlutWalks with teen girls. *Gender and Education*, *24*(3), 333–343.

Rofes, E. (2015). *Dry bones breathe: Gay men creating post-AIDS identities and cultures*. London: Routledge.

Sandset, T. (2019). PrEP at the margins: Toward a critically applied anthropology of Nordic PrEP access. *Somatosphere*. Retrieved from http://somatosphere.net/2019/prep -at-the-margins-toward-a-critically-applied-anthropology-of-nordic-prep-access.html/.

Sandset, T., & Wieringa, S. (2019). Impure policies: Controversy in HIV prevention and the making of evidence. *Critical Policy Studies*, 1–16.

Schackman, B. R., & Eggman, A. A. (2012). Cost–effectiveness of pre-exposure prophylaxis for HIV: A review. *Current Opinion in HIV and AIDS*, *7*(6), 587–592.

Singer, M. (1999). Anthropology and the politics of AIDS fatigue. *Anthropologie Newsletter*, *40*(3), 58.

Sontag, S. (1989). *AIDS and its metaphors* (Vol. 1). New York, NY: Farrar, Straus and Giroux.

Sontag, S. (2001). *Illness as metaphor and AIDS and its metaphors*. London: Macmillan.

Spieldenner, A. (2016). PrEP whores and HIV prevention: The queer communication of HIV pre-exposure prophylaxis (PrEP). *Journal of Homosexuality, 63*(12), 1685–1697.

Staley, Peter et al. (2015). Op-Ed: 10 Worst offenses of AIDS Healthcare Foundation's Michael Weinstein. *Plus Magazine*. Retrieved from https://www.hivplusmag.com/opi nion/2015/06/24/op-ed-10-worst-offenses-aids-healthcare-foundations-michael-wein stein.

Stern, Mark Joseph (2014). The enfant terrible of AIDS activism reaches a new low. *Slate*. Retrieved from https://slate.com/human-interest/2014/09/michael-weinstein-of-the -aids-healthcare-foundation-hates-truvada-don-t-listen-to-him.html.

The Lancet, H. I. V. (2015). PrEP: Why are we waiting? *The Lancet HIV, 2*(10), e401. doi:10.1016/S2352-3018(15)00185-X.

Treichler, P. A. (1999). *How to have theory in an epidemic: Cultural chronicles of AIDS*. Durham: Duke University Press.

UNAIDS. (2018). Miles to go—closing gaps, breaking barriers, righting injustices. 268.

Weinstein, Michael (2015). The war against prevention in *Business Wire*. Retrieved from https://www.businesswire.com/news/home/20150616006589/en/CORRECTING%C2 %A0and-REPLACING%C2%A0GRAPHIC-AHF-President-Calls-Attention-.

Wienmeyer, Richard (2014). Truvada: No substitute for responsible sex. *The Hastings Center*. Retrieved from https://www.thehastingscenter.org/truvada-no-substitute-for-responsible-sex/.

6   HIV both starts and stops with me
Health promotions, neoliberalism and responsibility

Introduction

While the end of AIDS and reaching epidemic control has been the subject of large international organizations and their strategies, at the end of the day, it is the individual subject that, more often than not, is targeted by prevention efforts. In this chapter, I want to explore some of the HIV prevention campaigns that have emerged recently in the wake of the drive to 'end AIDS'. Specifically, I want to focus on campaigns from the US and England which play on and use the very slogan of 'ending AIDS'. I do this in an effort to supplement and nuance the large and often technologically focused efforts of indicators, metrics and maps that we have seen in prior chapters. More importantly, I do this in an effort to analyze a long-standing hallmark in the history of the HIV epidemic, namely health promotions aimed at the public and, in particular, men who have sex with men. As a focal point of public health authorities, communities affected by HIV and scholarly interests, health promotions that have aimed at preventing HIV, reducing stigma and increasing awareness about the HIV epidemic have a varied and diverse history. For instance, the British Wellcome Trust has a collection of 3,000 digitalized HIV/AIDS posters collected from across the globe under the HIV epidemic.[1] The collection represents 99 countries and a staggering 94 languages. The Wellcome Trust Collections states, 'Thomas Hill, a then-Amsterdam based collector, with a personal interest in countercultures, recognised the historical significance of the posters as evidence of the worldwide crisis'. Since then, the Wellcome Trust Collection has grown and is an archive for the signifying epidemic that Paula Treichler so elegantly argued for. In the US, The National Institute for Health has a small online archive[2] driven by the rationale that 'the messages in these posters reveal how public health educators and activists see themselves and their audiences, and how they conceptualize disease and define normal behavior'. In taking the NIH's statement seriously, I want in this chapter to map how recent health promotions portray *what* HIV prevention is, *who* is targeted and *why*. Furthermore, I take the use of images in these campaigns to be a clear example of what the end of AIDS has come to signify in the new era of PrEP, ARVs and the drive to suppress viral load metrics to undetectable levels.

These two examples are but a small portion of the many past and ongoing HIV campaigns meant to inform, prevent and represent HIV/AIDS as a public health crisis. Moreover, with the narrative of the end of AIDS as an event that is within reach, a new iconology has emerged that is worth analyzing as a way of following up on how HIV is now being portrayed. In seeing these recent changes in the field of HIV prevention and treatment, there has been an increase once again in public health campaigns that focus in on delivering HIV preventive health information to the public and, in particular, to people who are considered to be at elevated risk of an HIV infection. This chapter argues that newer HIV prevention campaigns that focus on reaching the public with information on how to prevent HIV infections are mainly built upon the rationale of 'a neoliberal sexual actor' (Adam, 2016; Sandset, 2019; Thomann, 2018). Elsewhere, I have argued that in

> newer health promotions aimed at HIV prevention, the sexual actor being represented is predicated upon the tenets of a neoliberal subject wherein market choice, rational risk analysis, personal responsibility, and personal entrepreneurship is in focus. Secondly, these health promotions, while being both inclusive in terms of sexualities and racialized identities that are portrayed within them, they nevertheless are reminiscent of neoliberal ideals that may or may not be available for the people who are most vulnerable in terms of HIV risk.
>
> (Sandset, 2019:658).

I follow this up as a provocation to explore the HIV campaigns to be analyzed in this chapter. I am, however, aware that the notion of neoliberalism as a catchall phrase can gloss over as much as it is able to explain if we are not careful in laying out what we mean by this term (Flew, 2012; Venugopal, 2015), a point I will return to later. Furthermore, I also recognize that neoliberal notions of responsibility and its impact on health care is not the only logic operating within HIV discourses. In fact, as several scholars have noted, neoliberal ideals often work as a form of assimilation. This means that neo-liberal ideals and regimes of health care and subjectivation can co-exist or even thrive on the incorporation of marginalized and minority subject positions (Sandset, 2019:658). In fact, scholars such as Hardt and Negri (Hardt and Negri, 2000), Boltanski and Chiapello (Boltanski and Chiapello, 2005) and Nealon (Nealon, 2007) have pointed this out.

In applying this insight to the signifying epidemic in the era of 'the end of AIDS' we

> should be careful to align neo-liberalism with a regime that de facto excludes sexual minorities and other minority positions. Rather we should look carefully at the ways in which neo-liberalism, in fact, tries to play on and assimilate these subject positions in ways that seek to incorporate these as productive parts within neo-liberalism.
>
> (Sandset, 2019:568)

Part of this chapter will indeed show that this is the case in the health promotions analyzed.

This chapter seeks to underline that while many of the HIV prevention campaigns are both sex positive, inclusive and play less on fear and more on pleasure, there is nevertheless some potential pitfalls associated with an overt reliance on notions of market-driven choice, rational risk calculation and a form of sexual entrepreneurship. The potential pitfalls in these health promotions are that they might leave behind those who for whatever reasons cannot comply with or access these tenets. I recognize that no single health promotion can include every single aspect of the social, economic and cultural issues within the HIV epidemic. Nor can they, for that matter, include each and every group affected by HIV. I argue, however, that the increased reliance on biomedical interventions and the highlighting of neoliberal ideals within HIV preventive campaigns might, in the long run, lead to the most vulnerable becoming left behind, thereby increasing their vulnerability.

Finally, throughout this chapter, I will highlight the ways in which these new health promotions are part of the new biomedical push to end AIDS while also being part of an epidemic of signification. How we portray the end of AIDS matters I argue, and it is worth examining as part of the signifying epidemic. It can tell us about the signals being sent on *how* to end AIDS, *who* is to end AIDS and what forms of responsibility comes with this ending of AIDS. In the end, the analysis is not meant as a form of generalizable analysis of the representation of HIV prevention writ large on a global scale. Rather, I seek to engage with the forms of responsibility, actions and tensions that can be teased out from these images and HIV campaigns.

Responsibility both starts and stops with me: know your status and access drugs!

Following modern HIV treatment and prevention guidelines and aligning with the 90-90-90 targets set out by the UNAIDS, HIV prevention efforts in today's climate have increasingly focused on increasing HIV testing; for people who test positive, access to and retention in HIV care is the next step (Sidibé, 2014). Finally, the ultimate goal of HIV treatment (also now part of prevention) is for PLHIV to achieve suppressed viral load measurements. In so doing, PLHIV will live close to normal life expectancies, have fewer co-morbidities and become unable to transmit HIV onward (Cohen, 2011, Cohen et al., 2012). As such, growing numbers of HIV health promotions now focus direct attention on increased HIV testing uptakes, accessing and adhering to PrEP, and if tested positive, accessing and adhering to ARVs. Condom usage is still also part of this discourse but is increasingly supplemented with a biomedicalization of sexuality and HIV prevention through the focus on pharmaceuticals.

Another key aspect of current HIV health promotions is the focus on 'key populations'. UNAIDS, the CDC and other international health authorities have explicitly stated that to end AIDS, key populations must be reached with treatment and prevention programs (UNAIDS, 2018). Key populations are defined by the WHO's *Consolidated Guidelines on HIV Prevention, Diagnosis, Treatment and Care for Key Populations* as '1) men who have sex with men, 2) people who inject drugs, 3) people in prisons and other closed settings, 4) sex workers and 5) transgender people'(World Health Organization, 2017). In light of this, many health promotions today are directly aimed at key populations, such as MSM and transgender women. Yet as we shall see, this also masks and forecloses certain aspects of the HIV epidemic that risk leaving people behind on the road to an HIV-free generation.

As a way of providing a snapshot of the iconography and semiotic economy of HIV health promotions, I have chosen to work with a select set of such campaigns. The first from the US is called *Play Sure*.[3] The health promotion from England is called *It Starts with Me*.[4] *Play Sure* was rolled out in New York City (NYC) in 2015 as part of the city's ambitions to 'end AIDS' by s. Following the announcement of the mayor, Bill de Blasio, *Play Sure* was rolled out with a live event wherein de Blasio, as Thomann describes, was standing 'in front of a large screen that read "From Vision to Reality, #EndAIDSNYC2020"' (Thomann, 2018:1001). At the same event, de Blasio said, 'We are resolved to end this epidemic. We have the tools. We're committed to using them. There's no hesitation. There's no delay... the time is now to end the epidemic once and for all. It's as simple as that'. (Thomann, 2018:1001). Part of this plan was the scale-up of new PrEP programs which are part and parcel of NYC's 'ending the epidemic' plan. Another part was the introduction of the *Play Sure* health promotion, a promotion which is a social media marketing campaign which included posters on subways and buses as well as a website[5] and YouTube videos.[6] The health promotion focuses on the take-home message of 'be sure, play sure, stay sure' and uses the headline of 'Together we can stop the spread of HIV and other sexually transmitted infections (STIs)'.[7]

It should be noted that there are historical and contextual differences between various HIV preventive campaigns. Barring a genealogical analysis of the many HIV preventive campaigns and their relationship to pleasure and sex, I do want to note that there are historical, contextual and ideological differences between HIV preventive campaigns based on whether or not they are initiated by state-run public health actors, HIV activists, NGOs or pharmaceutical companies. Furthermore, geographical location of such campaigns is also crucial for the visual imagery used and the extent to which sexuality is portrayed. As such, I do not profess to offer here a generalizable analysis of current HIV preventive health promotions and their iconography. Rather, I want to tease out some inferences based on the aforementioned health promotions, their images and their textual 'take-home messages'.

Framing responsibility through choice: it starts with me

While I was a visiting scholar at UC Berkeley in 2018, I took a Bay Area Rapid Transit (BART) train from MacArthur station to 16th Street Mission station on my way to a café. On the BART ride, I suddenly noticed a poster for a clinical trial that was ongoing for injectable PrEP. The headline was, 'Show us yer cheeks, PrEP is a pill that prevents HIV. Could it also be a shot? Volunteer for a PrEP research study and help us find out'.[8] Above was a cartoon strip depicting four naked buttocks with reference to the headline 'Show us yer cheeks'. The poster immediately got my attention and I searched Google to find out more. As I was racing underground on my BART train, I learned that the clinical study was on the effects of long-lasting injectable PrEP conducted by Bridge HIV. Bridge HIV is, as they themselves note,

> a global leader in HIV prevention research, working with Bay Area and international communities to discover effective HIV prevention strategies. Operating as a clinical trials unit within the San Francisco Department of Public Health and affiliated with the University of California, San Francisco (UCSF), we conduct innovative research that guides global approaches in HIV prevention.[9]

While this in and of itself was interesting enough, what got my attention was thinking about *responsibility* in terms of who is to volunteer for these trials, who would benefit from them and ultimately who would benefit from the emergence of a long-lasting injectable. In starting this process, I started looking at various images of current HIV health promotions that soon led me to many of the photos and posters online for the *Play Sure* campaign. I had already become somewhat privy to the *Play Sure* initiative that was ongoing in NYC, but, in looking at these images, I started thinking through notions of risk, responsibility and what these images signified in relation to the notion of ending AIDS.

In the *Play Sure* campaign, the health promotion states that 'Together we can stop the spread of HIV and other sexually transmitted infections (STIs)'.[10] Through the slogan 'Be Sure, Play Sure, Stay Sure', the campaign plays on the notions of staying 'sure', that is mitigating risk and taking action to do so through HIV testing in order to 'be sure'; playing 'sure', the use of condoms and lube in order to 'play sure'; and, finally, staying 'sure' using PrEP or, if one is HIV-positive, then staying on treatment in order to 'stay sure'.[11] The line of argument is benign enough I argue, yet it also alludes to the points made by Diprose (Diprose, 2008) and Thomann (Thomann, 2018) that, within current HIV discourses of biomedicine and risk, there is a tendency to view the danger of an HIV infection as being omnipresent yet avoidable through the use of preventive technologies. Furthermore, throughout the entire 'chain' within this narrative, the possibility of an HIV infection is highlighted implicitly by the continual, personalized responsibility of 'being sure, playing sure and staying sure'.

Under the heading of 'Be Sure', to be 'sure' is to 'know your HIV status', and to 'know your STI status'. Specifically, to be sure is to get tested at least annually or, if you are an MSM or transgender person, every three to six months. This has also been highlighted by UNAIDS in a report entitled *Knowledge is power. Know your status, know your viral load.*[12] The UNAIDS states that

> An HIV test is a serious event with potentially serious outcomes. But no matter the result, the test provides vital information. A negative result is an

opportunity to take deliberate steps to prevent future acquisition through prevention methods tailored to that individual's risks. A positive test result—and a confirmatory diagnosis—is never welcome news, but for people living with HIV, it is a necessary first step towards a long and healthy life.[13]

HIV testing is important and is crucial in linking people to care and accessing treatment. Yet what is interesting is the individualizing focus on 'know *your* status' contrasted against the process which unfolds *after* an HIV test. A negative result does not mean the end of self-monitoring or risk calculation. Rather, a negative result actually *opens up* for an individualized evaluation of one's own risk for HIV and subsequent steps to access appropriate HIV preventive technologies. As such, the HIV test initiates a continual and almost omnipresent evaluation of one's own risk at all times.

This is also found in the *Play Sure* campaign. The webpage states, 'Getting tested and knowing your HIV status is the first step toward taking care of your health' and then goes on to note that 'If you test negative, you can learn about pre-exposure prophylaxis (PrEP) and other HIV prevention options'.[14] In a paradoxical fashion, a health promotion that plays on the idea of 'being sure' frames an HIV test as never enough, or rather, the risk of an HIV infection is almost omnipresent and only through continual monitoring and vigilance can one truly mitigate the risk of HIV. In a sense this is in line with the paradigm of anticipation in global health that Vincanne Adams et al. has written about (Adams et al., 2009). It is up to the individual to continually appraise, evaluate and anticipate HIV risks thus inhabiting both the present and potential futures, which can be anticipated or rather imagined at different levels of risk.

Pivoting back to the notion of responsibility and the *Play Sure* campaign, when promotion was rolled out in 2015, it was done so by a subsequent push in which the NYC Department of Health and Mental Hygiene also designed a *Play Sure* kit. The kit is framed as 'a case that allows you to easily and discreetly transport everything you need to practice safer sex'. While such kits can be appreciated as a way of giving individuals access to condoms, PrEP, and water based lubricants, Matthew Thomann reminds us that such kits can also be seen as a way of 'decentralizing biomedical prevention strategies, and taking them out of the clinic, putting them directly in the hand of the individual' (Thomann, 2018:1001). My argument here is that this can be read as a way of playing on market logics of choice, which is in turn predicated upon individuals being able to access these kits and evaluate risk through what is often seen as a form of 'rational actor theory'. HIV preventive tools have increasingly become mobile and transportable through 'at-home HIV testing kits' (Banda, 2015; Walensky and Paltiel, 2006) and 'widgets' that allow for HIV testing through smartphone apps (Draz et al., 2018). Other mobile technologies which take HIV out of the clinic can be seen in the ongoing development of apps that provide access to care and that alert PLHIV and PrEP users to take their medication;[15] and an ongoing study named the *PHAST Study*, which investigates how men who have sex with men can benefit from an app that will allow at-home HIV and STI testing as well as

PrEP.[16] One could argue that there is an entire subfield of HIV science dedicated to developing and analyzing HIV mobile and smartphone technology, some of them even playing on the concept of 'gamefication' (Hightow-Weidman et al., 2017; Muessig et al., 2015) to track PrEP adherence by providing a gaming experience that unlocks points and awards for 'playing' the app.[17] By taking HIV diagnosis and prevention out of the clinic, I argue that there is a certain decentralization at play at the same time as there is a market logic of choice and of individual responsibility at play. In order to make this argument clearer I want to clarify what I am here referring to by giving a brief account of neoliberalism in this setting.

A note on neoliberalism at the end of AIDS

As a model of rationality beyond the political economy of the state, neoliberalism invokes, enables and legitimizes practices such as managerialism, deregulation, efficiency, cost–benefit analysis, expanding various forms of entrepreneurial practices and privatization – all of which function in the interest of extending and disseminating values to all institutions and social actions (Giroux, 2008:590). This way of conceptualizing neoliberalism outside of its traditional associations with the state 'writ large' shows us that it is not just the state that is the target or rather the locus of neoliberal government, rather it is also people and their actions, their conduct. Following in the footsteps of Michel Foucault, recent efforts in connecting the dissemination of a neoliberal rationale embedded not just within the government of the state but also in the 'the conduct of men' (Foucault, 2007), neoliberalism can be seen as a set of 'epistemic commitments' (Sastry and Dutta, 2012). These epistemic commitments can be seen as a set of rationalities which have become what Pierre Bourdieu described as doxic or doxa (Bourdieu, 1977). This argues that the tenets of neoliberalism have become so embedded within Western societies that they are seen as 'common sense' or rather that this process describes an 'ensemble of fundamental beliefs of a field which do not need to express themselves through a formal dogma conscious of itself' (Sastry & Dutta, 2012:23). However, in specifying how this can be linked to health care and HIV prevention, we need to go the route of Michel Foucault in more detail.

First, we can note the theme of the neoliberal subject as an individual who 'invests' in himself/herself. This idea, so central to theories on human capital, will be brought into the analysis of the empirical material that is here. This notion of 'investing in oneself' as laid out by Foucault, is structured, according to Foucault, by its connection to the concept of homo economicus (Foucault, 2008:226). For Foucault, this means that man becomes within the neo-liberal frame of analysis, an entrepreneur of him/herself, that is 'the man of consumption, insofar as he consumes, is a producer. What does he produce? Well, quite simply, he produces his own satisfaction' (Foucault, 2008:226). In reading this, we might also briefly link this to how health promotions such as *Play Sure* and *It Starts with Me* indeed highlight the ways in which MSM can become consumers that consume preventive drugs or use preventive technologies in order to be both healthy *and* sexually satisfied. This seems very timely in relation to the ways in which people are targeted by these HIV preventive ads to invest in their health. By consuming a drug for PrEP, the subject produces his/her own (sexual) satisfaction, that is, the investiture of health, prophylactically, produces pleasure. One key aspect of this theory of neoliberal subjectification lies in the following quote from Foucault when he states that homo economicus 'as entrepreneur of himself, being for himself his own capital, being for himself his own producer, being for himself the source of [his] earnings' (Foucault, 2008:226). Extrapolated to the field of health care this form of subjectivity opens up for an understanding of the subject as not only responsible for his/her own health, but also that whatever choices are taken up by the subject in terms of health it can be read as an investment, something that will yield something back in return later on, a calculus of rationality wherein 'In sum, neoliberalism is about "[t]he application of the economic grid to social phenomena"' (McGuigan, 2014:229). This can clearly be seen in the continual focus on HIV testing; no matter the result, the HIV test is an investment that if negative will allow the subject to continue to evaluate HIV risk and take the necessary steps to 'stay sure'. If positive, then the subject must seek out care and treatment and ultimately strive to become undetectable as many scholars have written about (Alfonso et al., 2006; Cormier McSwiggin, 2017; Grace et al., 2015).

According to Foucault, governing in a neoliberal way, entails seeking to create an environment that influences the subject to make certain choices rather than others, i.e., that neoliberal thought imagines an actor that is situated within a 'milieu' or an 'environment' that gives shape to his/her conduct and choices, a key component in Foucault's notion of 'conduct of conduct' (Foucault, 2008). The strategy of creating healthy subjects by shaping the environments in which they make their (health) choices has been studied from a Foucauldian perspective by, for instance, Lars Thorup Larsen (Larsen & Stone, 2015). I seek to also show how notions of individual responsibility in the health promotions are not only underpinned by market logics of prevention or individual responsibility, but also to a large degree, play on pleasure and sexuality. I argue that these HIV prevention campaigns play on and create an environment wherein the sexual energies of the population are targeted by these ads and are shaped by playing on desire and pleasure rather than repressing these human emotions.

Sex, choice, prevention and the individual: playing sure to end AIDS

As I was looking at the many *Play Sure* images, browsing the campaign webpages and trying to connect the health promotion to broader issues in the narrative of ending AIDS, I came across several YouTube videos launched in connection with the campaign. One video struck me in particular in relationship to the ways in which the tensions between individual responsibility, market choice and sex and pleasure become evident.

In this video, we see a young Black man who connects with another man on an online hookup app. The viewer briefly sees the content of their conversation, as the young man types, 'I'll bring the [PrEP emoji], [condom emoji], [NYC Play Sure Kit emoji]'. This is followed by a female voice-over which says

> We all love to play, but we gotta play sure. So, whatever *your pleasure* or wherever you are, always be ready with the right combination protection that works for you. New York City has made it easy with the new NYC Play Sure Kit. Carry PrEP medications for HIV protection, HIV treatment, and condoms for added protection from HIV and other STIs. Or whatever *works best for you*. NYC plays sure. We're healthy and plan on staying that way.[18]

By looking at the words that I have put in italics, I argue that we can see how the *Play Sure* health promotion indeed plays on rhetorical tropes that I have argued previously are in line with what has been identified as neo-liberal ideals of market choice, individual responsibility and the decentralization of health care from the state to the individual. In this case, the promo video invokes the notions of fusing individual desires with rhetoric that also states that the individual can choose where and when to stay protected and with what kind of protective technologies, be that PrEP, condoms and/or using lube. Yet the video does not shy away from issues of sex and pleasure, indeed it utilizes these aspects to precisely play on these issues in fostering a 'milieu' as Foucault perhaps would have called it. Finally, there is also a strong degree of *anticipation* and *preemption* deployed. While there is a great deal of focus on the individual and his/her responsibility to *choose* the right protective technology that works for them, this is connected to the anticipation of sex. 'Always be ready' seems radically different from the idea that the best prevention for HIV is abstinence. On the contrary, the video seems to suggest that sex and pleasure can happen almost anywhere and at anytime, yet always also suggesting that there is an inherent risk of HIV and STI infections, hence the need to carry protection.

Another instance of this is the second *Play Sure* video related to the campaign. Here the viewer first sees a man and a woman sitting on a sofa kissing and caressing each other while the setting seems to be a house party with funk music playing. The viewer is then addressed by the woman who says 'we play sure with PrEP and condoms' followed by a narrator who informs that 'PrEP is an easy-to-use pill that reduces your risk of an HIV infection by over 90 percent.' The video then cuts to two African-American men who hold each other while at the same house party. One of the men addresses the camera by saying 'we play sure with PrEP, HIV treatment, and condoms', after which the narrator of the video informs the viewer that 'HIV treatment can lower your viral load to undetectable levels and keep your partner safe'.[19]

Once again, the *Play Sure* ads conjure up notions of choice, individual responsibility and the notion that there is a customizable form of HIV prevention for you if you take the time to make the right choice that fits you. The emphasis in these voice-overs is on the responsibility of the individual to carry the proper protective technologies at all times as 'one never knows' what a sexual encounter might lead to. HIV risk is mitigated by this kit, which further shows the decentralization of responsibility away and out of the clinic while also indicating a certain amount of choice for the individual, a market logic of 'choosing whatever works for you'. The videos can be read as metonyms for the entire neoliberal sexual actor; risk is omnipresent but can be mitigated by personal responsibility which has to do with making the right choice in terms of preventive technologies which in turn moves responsibility away from the state or the clinic and onto the individual. Linking this to the work of Foucault, these videos both build upon an idea of the subject as being an individual that invests in their own health by 'staying safe' while, at the same time, also create an environment wherein the desires of the subjects (i.e., one of their motivational factors, that is sexuality) is played on actively and openly as a way of enticing the subject into investing in both sex and prevention.

The customization of HIV prevention is highly individualized and the environment that is being created is one which seeks to influence the subject to make certain choices rather than others, in this case, either by using PrEP, ART, condoms or a combination of the three. However, what is striking is that this environment and this 'nudging' of the individual toward these modalities is being conducted through an alignment of sex and pleasure, rather than disciplinary repression of these issues.

Sex and pleasure, risk and responsibility and a present tense, which is always inhabited by anticipating the future. A present that always must anticipate the risky future, seems to emerge in these health promotions. Yet the biomedicalization of sexuality and the mitigation of risk by preventive technologies seem to tell us, the viewers, that sex is okay as long as we monitor our risks, choose the right preventive technologies and are able to anticipate our futures.

In the context of health and the intersection between a neoliberal actor and a neoliberal society, assumptions about health often times starts out from the assumption that (1) health is largely an individual and private responsibility, (2) that ill health is caused by allocative and technical inefficiencies and (3) that health can be improved through, for example, cost-effective interventions and the increase of market forces in health services so as to increase choice of treatment and care (Sastry & Dutta, 2012:24). As Barry Adam remarks in relation to the idea of the neoliberal actor in HIV prevention:

> The contract-making citizen presumed by liberal democracies and the choice-making consumer of the capitalist marketplace circulate through the 'health belief models' and 'theories of reasoned action' that take up so much attention in health research and promotion. From defensive driving to smoking cessation, the rational man—and it is often a gendered conception—avoids perils to health because he seeks naturally to maximize his own longevity and wellbeing while avoiding risk. In the marketplace of life, the rational actor is a conscious, informed calculator of risk and gain.
>
> (Adam, 2006:169)

Adam makes an important point and that is that these neoliberal dictums now increasingly have come to define the ways in which the subject is seen as being in relation to his/her own body and health and in this context, HIV prevention and the individual's unique responsibility of doing their part in 'ending AIDS'.

Pivoting back to the *Play Sure* campaign, I want to think through a set of posters that were launched as part of the campaign. As I was digging through the iconography and images of the many current HIV preventive campaigns – the *Play Sure* campaign included – I started to think through how intimacy and pleasure intersected and were used in this campaign. For instance, one of the ads contains the imagery of two men holding each other with the tagline 'Be HIV sure. One night can change your HIV status. Be safe, be sure. And get tested frequently'.[20] Once again, we see the continual focus on the omnipresence of HIV as a risk that needs to be mitigated through continual surveillance and mediated through HIV testing. Another of the *Play Sure* posters depict two African-American men dressed in jeans and both of them wearing tank tops. One is kissing the other on the cheek while the man being kissed is depicted as laughing. Underneath the slogan is 'We play sure. PrEP + HIV treatment + condoms'.[21] While the *Play Sure* website is much more explicit in its individualized focus, the posters contain a much more 'we' focused imagery. However, they do share the continual focus on biomedical technologies of prevention and the importance of continual testing, consumption of biopharma and condom usage. Risk is also an element that seems omnipresent even though it can be overcome by testing and consumption of PrEP or ART.

Linking the aforementioned empirical material back to the notion of a neoliberal subject that invests in his/herself, one could state that the rollout of the Play Sure Kit, in fact, is part and parcel of this type of investment. By buying or procuring such kits the individual injunction seems to be that as long as the subject invests both time and money in terms of taking, for instance, PrEP, the subject invests in staying healthy. However, perhaps more novel in this setting, he/she also invests in their sex life thus the investment of PrEP and 'staying sure' is also an investment into a sexual economy of pleasure. Put slightly differently this sort of neo-liberal investment into the personal health of the individual is also made possible by the incorporation of desire and pleasure as part of the investment process. Contrary to the older tropes, wherein the investment of health was made through abstinence, monogamy and condom usage, these new health ads, in fact, invoke pleasure as a way of investing in one's own health.

However, broader societal drivers of the epidemic are left out, and no mention of syndemic vectors are mentioned, thus leaving out issues such as poverty, homelessness and mental health as important factors. Not only does this leave out important vectors for prevention within the epidemic, such as clean needle programs and methadone treatment programs, but it also leaves out the people who deal with these issues. While we should acknowledge that these campaigns have moved away from the earlier focus of the 'ABCs of HIV', that is, abstinence, being faithful (monogamous) and using condoms (Dworkin & Ehrhardt, 2007), and now allow for a more sex-positive outlook on HIV/AIDS, there is a configuration of the individual's responsibility to stay both sure and safe in these ads. It is important to highlight that while these health promotions are indeed sex-positive, inclusive and, to a large degree, borrow tropes that convey a message wherein HIV is not the 'doom and gloom' of older health promotions, they nevertheless can be seen as representing a potential problematic turn in HIV prevention. While we should acknowledge that not every health promotion can target all of the different groups affected by HIV, the omission of syndemic drivers, such as drug use and the chem sex scene, discrimination either based on homophobia or racism and psychological stressors such as depression, isolation and anxiety are problematic. The danger is not the scale-up of health promotions such as these nor the rollout of ART, testing and PrEP regimes; rather the problem might be that if these modes of configuring and framing the subject become doxic themselves, this might undermine focus on systemic drivers of the epidemic as well as the syndemic drivers of HIV risk. These health promotions, I argue, reconfigure the PrEP user within a framework which relies heavily on a notion of a neoliberal sexual actor and associates PrEP with personal responsibility, a free market of options and making a rational choice for one's health.

As Thomann states,

> If these campaigns are any indication of the configuration of the individual who is 'to end AIDS', then we can expect more health promotions that focus on the neoliberal sexual citizen as one who is a 'pre-emptive patient-consumer' who is made responsible not through risk avoidance but rather through the consumption of biomedical interventions.
>
> (Thomann, 2018:9)

Furthermore, if this configuration of the sexual citizen is the one which will dominate in the coming years, the danger is that those who do not have access to these biomedical preventive technologies, who cannot afford them, or who cannot adhere to them for whatever reason – be that transient homelessness, mental health issues, or economic issues wherein income and insurance are unstable – will be 'left behind'.

Disciplining for pleasure: anticipating, pre-emption, planning and pleasure

Thinking through the issues of how key populations are targeted by HIV preventive health promotions and, in connection to this, how responsibility, health and pleasure are framed in rhetoric that plays on the end of AIDS, I quickly started to look around me for these kinds of images. In my native Norway, in the capital of Oslo, the visibility of the HIV epidemic is all but non-existent. I haven't seen a billboard, poster or advertisement for anything that has to do with HIV in a long time. The HIV epidemic in Norway is comparatively small with 6468 people who are living with HIV; of these, 4382 are men and 2086 are women.[22] The epidemic is mainly concentrated amongst MSM men, immigrants who are

HIV-positive prior to coming to Norway and a smaller fraction of heterosexual men who become HIV-positive while abroad. In this milieu, the HIV epidemic is by and large 'out of sight, out of mind' for the broader public in Oslo.

However, in the Bay Area, comprising San Francisco, Oakland, South San Francisco, Marin County and, to a certain degree, San Jose, the story is different. Much of the time doing research for this book was spent in San Francisco and here HIV is more visible and more tangible. Walking through San Francisco one day, I noticed a PrEP commercial produced by the San Francisco Department of Public Health (SFDPH). The poster had the headline 'Our sexual revolution' with the subtext of 'PrEP is a pill for people who are HIV-negative. It protects you from HIV. PrEP is safe and effective condoms prevent other STDs'. The imagery in the background was of four men of different ethnicities as well as an African-American woman.[23] This got me thinking about what this sexual revolution heralded by PrEP was. I personally knew several people who were on PrEP and who felt that PrEP was a drug that had made their intimate and sexual lives easier and, above all, had lifted a lot of the mental anguish of constantly fearing an HIV infection. In short, many of the people I personally knew would perhaps have agreed that PrEP was a form of sexual revolution.

Looking at this poster piqued my interest in the visual and textual messaging that PrEP advertisements were delivering. In particular I wanted to follow up on the notion of 'the revolutionary'. For me, sexual revolution held connotations of radical change, the 1970s, women's liberation and 'free love'. PrEP, it seems, inserted itself into this discourse, although as I have shown in the previous chapter, not without various forms of backlash. There is one particularly telling and, I argue, novel feature of many of the PrEP advertisements: the trope of 'freedom' and 'being in the moment'. I seek to tease out some of the tensions in PrEP promotion and what they can tell us about personal responsibility and the individualization of ending AIDS.

I found two posters that are particularly illustrative for my focus on the notion of PrEP as revolutionary and liberating: one is an Australian PrEP promotion called 'I'm Ending HIV', sponsored by New South Wales campaign *PositiveLifeNSW*; the other is from the SFDPH *Getting to Zero* campaign.[24]

In the first poster from the NSW *Ending AIDS* campaign, we see two men who are both bare-chested and framed in a posture of intimacy. Both have their eyes closed and are frozen in place as in the moment before a kiss or, perhaps, an intimate touch. The accompanying text states, 'Be in the moment. A once-a-day pill that keeps you HIV-negative'. In the SFDPH poster, we see two Latino men in bed, one is resting his head on the chest of the other while both are bare-chested. The two men are looking directly into the camera with the following text under the image: 'Get liberated. Take it' in bold letters. Underneath, it says 'PrEP is a pill that prevents HIV. Take it once a day. Stay negative'.

While playing on pleasure and the freedom to enjoy sex virtually whenever the moment arises, the ads are still part of the test and treatment paradigms as seen through the 'linguistic equation' of 'test often', 'treat early' and 'stay safe' that will 'end HIV in 2020'. A lingering 'responsibilization' of health also remains here. A statement in the top left corner of the first ad says 'I'm ending HIV', a clear individualization of HIV and a reminder that ending HIV is a personal responsibility. As such, the imagery and written messages in the image still display the disciplinary logic of risk minimization in their emphasis on contagion, testing and treatment. However, contrary to a focus that only highlights risk and contagion, these campaigns *also* speak to such tropes as pleasure and sex. The slogan 'be in the moment' points to an almost unlimited access to pleasure and sex if only one commits to PrEP.

These ads specifically target MSM, and while targeted HIV prevention campaigns are crucial in HIV-preventive work, other scholars have drawn attention to how PrEP discourses might unintentionally exclude other groups possibly needing PrEP (Amico & Bekker, 2019). The argument advanced is that, although targeted campaigns like those above are important, they also risk reifying and stigmatizing PrEP use as accessible *only* to people in certain 'risk groups', thus discounting those in possible need of PrEP as an added protective technology. For example, women in the USA might come to view PrEP as an option for gay men only (Amico & Bekker, 2019:e318). The emphasis on risk as a strategy for ensuring target groups' procurement, enrollment and adherence has been termed a 'loss-framed' approach to HIV prevention (Amico & Bekker, 2019:e317). While 'loss-framed' or 'risk-based' prevention has been successful, scholars have nevertheless highlighted the need for campaigns that foreground *protection rather than risk*, particularly as a means of addressing individuals who do not perceive themselves as being 'at risk'. Contrary to risk-based ads, whose PrEP messages might inadvertently miss, or even deter, large portions of the very population that could benefit from PrEP (Amico & Bekker, 2019:e318), the pleasure- and protection-focused ads analyzed here might attract people who do not see themselves as being 'at risk' but who want to 'be in the moment' *while* being protected.

We can link this to the insights that a key reason why behavioral interventions have failed to check the HIV epidemic is that in so-called 'hot moments' of decision-making, some ignore their knowledge regarding preventive measures (Grant & Koester, 2016:4). For example, condom usage might not be possible due to personal preferences, the lack of a condom when needed, or such factors as a sense of safety or the influence of drugs, which might cause a person to evaluate risk differently (Grant & Koester, 2016:4). As such, PrEP in so-called 'cold moments' of risk evaluation (Grant & Koester, 2016:5) allows one to experience unmitigated pleasure and have safe sex without the need for prior consideration. One could translate the above poster's reference to 'being in the moment' as the freedom from having to calculate risks in the heat of such a moment, as Grant and Koester note. Instead, PrEP allows one to calculate the risk of potential 'hot moments', whereas condom usage must be negotiated in the very heat of them. Kane Race has described this as 'the paradox of the planned slipup' (Race, 2016; Race, 2017). As Race states,

> PrEP asks HIV-negative men not only to *acknowledge* but also take systematic, prescribed, coordinated and involved action against a risk that one

may not be inclined to acknowledge so readily. Or against a risk that *may* be acknowledged at some level, but that is rationalised as *not much* of a risk [...] something that happens spontaneously, irregularly, or in the heat of the moment.

(Race, 2017:106)

My focus here is on the temporal dimension of what Race alludes to, the notion of *anticipation, calculation and pre-emption*, which stands in an intricate relationship in the aforementioned campaigns with *the spontaneous, the pleasurable and the playful.*

This observation hints at the ways in which PrEP consumption for pleasure challenges seeing gay men's engagement with various forms of biomedical treatment and prevention technologies as deterministic, thus advancing the logics of neoliberalism. Rather, as the scholarship of Kane Race and Martin Holt emphasize, the co-production of biomedical technologies and gay and bisexual male (GBM) communities is often creative and entails the entanglements of drugs, HIV preventive technologies and pleasure (Race, 2016; Race, 2015b; Race, 2015a; Holt, 2015; Holt, 2014).

PrEP allows one to defer risk calculations to the moments before, or outside of, the sexual encounter itself. This does not relieve the subject of risk calculations or disciplinary demands; after all, adhering to PrEP is disciplinary in an almost literal sense, since the individual must stick to consuming a measured daily dose of PrEP. However, the well-balanced subject in this analysis relegates risk calculations to other times and other spaces than those dictated by, say, condom usage. The well-balanced subject that figures in these ads balances pleasure and planning – risk calculation and desire – by consuming PrEP in 'cold moments'. Risk calculation becomes a *pre-emptive* strategy that allows the PrEP user to 'be in the moment', as the poster so vividly states.

This also touches upon rationales for starting PrEP. Grant and Koester note that PrEP users report that their decision to start taking the drug was based not only on the safety factor but also on the increased pleasure that they would be able to experience (Grant & Koseter, 2016:5–7). Other factors include adaptability, a sense of empowerment, reduction of mental stress and psychological anxiety as well as the fostering of communal bonds of love and care (Grant & Koseter, 2016:5–7). However, as a corrective to this optimistic framing of PrEP, it should also be noted that PrEP has also been an object of controversy wherein PrEP was linked to 'promiscuity' and seen as a 'fun pill' for people who do not want to be 'responsible'. A case in point is Pawson and Grov's study on attitudes toward PrEP amongst MSM in New York, where the authors show how PrEP becomes a contentious issue as well as an object wherein some are deemed to be 'deserving' PrEP users versus 'undeserving' PrEP users (Pawson & Grov, 2018:1396).

The imagery of these ads plays on intimacy, the biomedical consumption of pharmaceuticals and the idea of liberation, which seems to take three forms: a temporal liberation from the endless imperative to evaluate risk in every sexual encounter without PrEP, a liberation from the fear of HIV infection and, finally, the liberty to be intimate without anxiety. Once again, Robert Grant and Kimberley Koester highlight how emerging ethnographic research and surveys show that people go on PrEP for reasons other than simply ensuring that they can practice riskier sex with a greater number of partners (Grant & Koester, 2016:6). Even people with a limited number of partners report that their principal reason for taking PrEP is the comfort of knowing that they are 'safe' and protected, a factor that points to psychological aspects of PrEP that extend beyond unmediated pleasure and sex (Grant & Koester, 2016:6). While these PrEP commercials do not convey the message that 'anything goes', their message does transform and insert discipline into a new temporal logic of pre-emption, planning and subsequent pleasure, as PrEP usage and health ads, unlike condom usage and perhaps also condom promotions, are, after all, based on an acknowledgment of the ever-present risk of HIV. As such, the introspective realization that one will engage in risky sexual activities indeed mediates a decision to start taking PrEP. In this framework, the well-balanced subject is someone who negotiates pleasure and risk through pre-emption and planning, that is, by striking a balance between the aspiration to have pleasurable, condomless sex in the future and the discipline required to adhere to a daily regimen of PrEP pills. PrEP, then, disciplines through rational planning and through a perpetual self-control and introspection in which the individual plans ahead. There is, of course, also an underlying rationale of risk and discipline embedded within PrEP campaigns, such as those relating to the fact that the PrEP *guidelines* themselves are often bound to the fact that to qualify for PrEP to begin with, the subject must be 'at risk'. Contrary to these ads, wherein risk is less an element of the iconology, being *screened* for PrEP relies, to a large degree, on acknowledging sexual risky behavior and thus being interpellated as 'being at risk'.

This last point is crucial for our contribution to both the analysis of how biomedicalization within HIV research can be interpreted on the basis of PrEP as well as the conceptual issue of the relationship between discipline and security. First, PrEP introduces a new temporal axis within HIV prevention, which we analyzed through the lenses of discipline and security. The disciplinary axis can be said to be formed through each individual's obligation to take PrEP *before* and *after* sexual encounters. The security axis constitutes, in turn, the temporality opened up by one's adhering to PrEP and thus allowing desire and pleasure to come to the fore and risks to be minimized. At the level of the exposed population, PrEP creates another kind of temporality analyzable from the standpoint of security – the infection rate as something calculable over time and space.

While pleasure and sex have already figured in earlier HIV prevention campaigns that focused on condom usage, condom usage as a means of biomedicalization does not create the same sort of temporality that we have identified. Biomedicalization of sexuality and pleasure through the temporality of PrEP is not only driven, as Persson has stated, by 'an ambition to 'transform' and 'normalize' such phenomena and, in the process, transform bodies, identities and socialities' (Persson, 2013:1066). In fact, the biomedicalization of sexuality and pleasure by means of PrEP institutes a new health prevention temporality that can be understood as an integration of discipline and security. This last point regarding the transformation of temporality in health prevention is our key contribution to the growing field of sociological research exploring the evolving biomedicalization of HIV prevention. PrEP *anticipates* risk: it prepares for it and simultaneously mitigates it. Indeed, the very fact that one takes PrEP in 'cold moments' of introspection (Grant & Koester, 2016) and thus pre-emptively anticipates risky sex distinguishes PrEP from a strict disciplinary regime. Accordingly, the premise of the campaign could be condensed into this mutual condition: without risk management, no pleasure; and, conversely, without pleasure, no effective risk management.

The key differences that this well-balanced subject manifests in comparison to previous subject positions is the constant balancing act that PrEP demands: pre-emption and planning at 'cold moments' in anticipation of future moments where the subject can 'get liberated' and simply enjoy.

Notes

1 See the collection; https://wellcomelibrary.org/collections/digital-collections/aids-posters/
2 See the NIH archive; https://www.nlm.nih.gov/exhibition/visualculture/target.html
3 See the New York City based 'Play Sure' health promotion; https://www1.nyc.gov/site/doh/health/health-topics/playsure.page
4 See It Starts with Me; https://www.hivpreventionengland.org.uk/it-starts-with-me/
5 See the Play Sure website; https://www1.nyc.gov/site/doh/health/health-topics/play sure.page
6 See the YouTube videos here; https://www.youtube.com/watch?v=SZU6nibG35s, https://www.youtube.com/watch?v=RjfMj3FQULk, https://www.youtube.com/watch?v=W3ErsNQiZUA
7 See the webpage; https://www1.nyc.gov/site/doh/health/health-topics/hiv-besure-pla ysure-staysure.page
8 A Google image search will provide two examples of the poster; https://www.google .com/search?biw=1280&bih=603&tbm=isch&sxsrf=ACYBGNQdQpPr4l7S3rp8drvc PrxqCFXK-Q%3A1578494176566&sa=1&ei=4OgVXtiVIpWFwPAPgpul0AY&q =BART+HIV+posters&oq=BART+HIV+posters&gs_l=img.3...4544.7257..7564...0 .0..0.68.877.16......0....1..gws-wiz-img.......35i39j0i67j0j0i131j0i30j0i19j0i8i30.vdZ45 BFkwgs&ved=0ahUKEwjYhbKFnfTmAhWVAhAIHYJNCWoQ4dUDCAY&uact=5 #imgrc=ZsG604WhibjRCM:
9 See Bridge HIV; https://helpfighthiv.org/who-we-are/
10 See the Play Sure webpage; https://www1.nyc.gov/site/doh/health/health-topics/hiv-besure-playsure-staysure.page
11 See the Play Sure webpage; https://www1.nyc.gov/site/doh/health/health-topics/hiv-besure-playsure-staysure.page
12 See the document at UNAIDS; https://www.unaids.org/en/resources/documents/2018/ knowledge-is-power-report
13 See the document at UNAIDS; https://www.unaids.org/en/resources/documents/2018/ knowledge-is-power-report
14 See the webpage; https://www1.nyc.gov/site/doh/health/health-topics/hiv-be-hiv-sure .page
15 See HIV.gov for an entire list of mobile applications that focus on HIV prevention, care and treatment; https://www.hiv.gov/topics/mobile

16 See Bridge HIV's webpage for the study; https://helpfighthiv.org/our-research/
17 See the article on the P3 app (Prepared, Protected and Empowered); https://www.hiv
    .gov/blog/prep-there-s-app
18 See the video in full; https://www.youtube.com/watch?v=W3ErsNQiZUA
19 See the video in full; https://www.youtube.com/watch?v=RjfMj3FQULk
20 See the poster; https://www.thebody.com/article/new-york-citys-new-hiv-awareness-
    campaign-shows-in
21 See the poster and the campaign; https://desireekennedyproductions.wordpress.com/20
    15/12/15/i-bet-by-now-you-have-seen-the-nyc-plays-sure-campaign-on-the-subway/
22 See the Norwegian Center for Disease Control; https://hivnorge.no/wp-content/uploads
    /2019/03/Hivarsoppgjor-2018.pdf
23 See the poster at the 'Our Sexual Revolution' webpage; https://oursexualrevolution
    .org/
24 For the Australian health promotion see, https://endinghiv.org.au/blog/is-prep-for-you
    -campaign/. For the SFDPH campaign see the poster at Social Marketing, http://www
    .socialmarketing.com/campaign/get_liberated

References

Adam, B. D. (2016). Neoliberalism, masculinity, and HIV risk. *Sexuality Research and Social Policy*, *13*(4), 321–329.

Adams, V., Murphy, M., & Clarke, A. E. (2009). Anticipation: Technoscience, life, affect, temporality. *Subjectivity*, *28*(1), 246–265.

Alfonso, V., Geller, J., Bermbach, N., Drummond, A., & Montaner, J. S. (2006). Becoming a. treatment success: what helps and what hinders patients from achieving and sustaining undetectable viral loads. *AIDS Patient Care and STDs*, *20*(5), 326–334.

Amico, K. R., & Bekker, L.-G. (2019). Global PrEP roll-out: Recommendations for programmatic success. *The Lancet HIV*, *6*(2), e137–e140.

Banda, J. (2015). Rapid home HIV testing: Risk and the moral imperatives of biological citizenship. *Body & Society*, *21*(4), 24–47.

Boltanski, L., & Chiapello, E. (2005). The new spirit of capitalism. *International Journal of Politics, Culture, and Society*, *18*(3–4), 161–188.

Bourdieu, P. (1977). *Outline of a theory of practice*. Cambridge: Cambridge university Press.

Cohen, J. (2011). *HIV treatment as prevention*. American Association for the Advancement of Science.

Cohen, M. S., Mccauley, M., & Gamble, T. R. (2012). HIV treatment as prevention and HPTN 052. *Current Opinion in HIV and AIDS*, *7*(2), 99.

Cormier Mcswiggin, C. (2017). Moral adherence: HIV treatment, undetectability, and stigmatized viral loads among Haitians in South Florida. *Medical Anthropology*, *36*(8), 714–728.

Diprose, R. (2008). Biopolitical technologies of prevention. *Health Sociology Review*, *17*(2), 141–150.

Draz, M. S., Kochehbyoki, K. M., Vasan, A., Battalapalli, D., Sreeram, A., Kanakasabapathy, M. K. … Shafiee, H. (2018). DNA engineered micromotors powered by metal nanoparticles for motion based cellphone diagnostics. *Nature Communications*, *9*(1), 4282.

Dworkin, S. L., & Ehrhardt, A. A. (2007). Going beyond 'ABC' to include 'GEM': Critical reflections on progress in the HIV/AIDS epidemic. *American Journal of Public Health*, *97*(1), 13–18.

Flew, T. (2012). Michel Foucault's the Birth of biopolitics and contemporary neo-liberalism debates. *Thesis Eleven, 108*(1), 44–65.

Foucault, M. (2007). *Security, territory, population: Lectures at the Collège de France, 1977–78*. Berlin: Springer.

Foucault, M. (2008). *The birth of biopolitics: Lectures at the Collège de France, 1978–1979*. Berlin: Springer.

Giroux, H. A. (2008). Beyond the biopolitics of disposability: Rethinking neoliberalism in the New Gilded Age. *Social Identities, 14*(5), 587–620.

Grace, D., Chown, S. A., Kwag, M., Steinberg, M., Lim, E., & Gilbert, M. (2015). Becoming 'undetectable': Longitudinal narratives of gay men's sex lives after a recent HIV diagnosis. *AIDS Education and Prevention, 27*(4), 333–349.

Grant, R. M., & Koester, K. A. (2016). What people want from sex and preexposure prophylaxis. *Current Opinion in HIV and AIDS, 11*(1), 3–9.

Hardt, M., & Negri, A. (2000). *Empire*. Cambridge, MA: Harvard University Press.

Hightow-Weidman, L. B., Muessig, K. E., Bauermeister, J. A., Legrand, S., & Fiellin, L. E. (2017). The future of digital games for HIV prevention and care. *Current Opinion in HIV and AIDS, 12*(5), 501.

HIV/AIDS, J. U. N. P. O. & HIV/AIDS, J. U. N. P. O. (2014). *90-90-90: An ambitious treatment target to help end the AIDS epidemic*. Geneva: UNAIDS.

Holt, M. (2014). Gay men's HIV risk reduction practices: The influence of epistemic communities in HIV social and behavioral research. *AIDS Education and Prevention, 26*(3), 214–223.

Holt, M. (2015). Configuring the users of new HIV-prevention technologies: The case of HIV pre-exposure prophylaxis. *Culture, Health and Sexuality, 17*(4), 428–439.

Larsen, L. T., & Stone, D. (2015). Governing health care through free choice: Neoliberal reforms in Denmark and the United States. *Journal of Health Politics, Policy and Law, 40*(5), 941–970.

Mcguigan, J. (2014). The neoliberal self. *Culture Unbound: Journal of Current Cultural Research, 6*(1), 223–240.

Muessig, K. E., Nekkanti, M., Bauermeister, J., Bull, S., & Hightow-Weidman, L. B. (2015). A systematic review of recent smartphone, Internet and Web 2.0 interventions to address the HIV continuum of care. *Current HIV/AIDS Reports, 12*(1), 173–190.

Nealon, J. (2007). *Foucault beyond Foucault: Power and its intensifications since 1984*. Palo Alto, CA: Stanford University Press.

Pawson, M., & Grov, C. (2018). 'It's just an excuse to slut around'. gay and bisexual mens' constructions of HIV pre-exposure prophylaxis (Pr EP) as a social problem. *Sociology of Health and Illness, 40*(8), 1391–1403.

Persson, A. (2013). Non/infectious corporealities: Tensions in the biomedical era of 'HIV normalisation'. *Sociology of Health and Illness, 35*(7), 1065–1079.

Race, K. (2015a). 'Party and play': Online hook-up devices and the emergence of PNP practices among gay men. *Sexualities, 18*(3), 253–275.

Race, K. (2015b). Speculative pragmatism and intimate arrangements: Online hook-up devices in gay life. *Culture, Health and Sexuality, 17*(4), 496–511.

Race, K. (2016). Reluctant objects: Sexual pleasure as a problem for HIV biomedical prevention. *GLQ: A Journal of Lesbian and Gay Studies, 22*(1), 1–31.

Race, K. (2017). *The gay science: Intimate experiments with the problem of HIV*. London: Routledge.

Sandset, T. (2019). 'HIV Both Starts and Stops with Me': Configuring the neoliberal sexual actor in HIV prevention. *Sexuality and Culture, 23*, 657–673.

Sastry, S., & Dutta, M. J. (2012). Public health, global surveillance, and the 'emerging disease' worldview: A postcolonial appraisal of PEPFAR. *Health Communication, 27*(6), 519–532.

Sidibé, M. (2014). 90-90-90: A transformative agenda to leave no one behind. Hanoi, Vietnam. UNAIDS. https://www.unaids.org/sites/default/files/media_asset/20141025_SP_EXD_Vietnam_launch_of_909090_en.pdf

Thomann, M. (2018). 'On December 1, 2015, sex changes. Forever': Pre-exposure prophylaxis and the pharmaceuticalisation of the neoliberal sexual subject. *Global Public Health, 13*(18), 1–10.

UNAIDS. (2018). Miles to go—closing gaps, breaking barriers, righting injustices. 268.

Venugopal, R. (2015). Neoliberalism as concept. *Economy and Society, 44*(2), 165–187.

Walensky, R. P., & Paltiel, A. D. (2006). Rapid HIV testing at home: Does it solve a problem or create one? *Annals of Internal Medicine, 145*(6), 459–462.

World Health Organization (2017). Consolidated guidelines on HIV prevention, diagnosis, treatment and care for key populations, 2014. Retrieved from http://apps. who. int/iris/bitstream/10665/246200/1/9789241511124-eng. pdf.

7 The category is: Suppress! Disclose! Survive! 'Positive living' in health promotions for people living with HIV in the era of the end of AIDS

> *I've buried more friends in the last year than any of you can count! And when it's all over who knows how many of us will be left?*
> — Pray Tell (Billy Porter, Pose, Season 1, Episode 6 'Love is the Message')

Returning to Oslo, Norway after my research stay in San Francisco, I soon found myself watching the HBO series *Pose*. Set in the late 1980s and early 1990s, the show focuses on a group of transgender women, gay and queer men of color in New York at the height of the AIDS crisis and their lives. A primary focus of the show is the space of drag balls and *vogue* dancing popularized by the artist, Madonna, through her song titled 'Vogue'. The show empathically shows how these individuals navigate living in an era wherein the AIDS epidemic was decimating the LGBTQI communities of New York. Yet the FX drama also shows resilience, love and community; and while HIV/AIDS is not the primary focus of the show, the backdrop of the epidemic is always there, hidden, then emerging only to recede to the background as a revenant.

This section's subtitle is inspired by the show's opening line 'The category is: Live! Work! Pose!' narrated by the character Pray Tell (played by Billy Porter). Focusing on HIV health promotions that address living with HIV, I seek to highlight three 'categories' that recur in the era of ending AIDS for PLHIV. Those categories are achieving viral load suppression, disclosing HIV status in order to decrease stigma around living with HIV and surviving through ARV adherence and healthy living.

If in the above we have seen the configuration of a sort of neoliberal sexual actor who seeks to optimize pleasure while at the same time seeking to choose a preventive option that is *just right* for themselves, then health promotions aimed at PLHIV follow a similar trajectory, I argue. In fact, in many of the current HIV health promotions, there are no longer clear-cut distinctions between addressing people who are HIV-negative and PLHIV.

In the following, I take a few snapshots of health promotions that are addressed to PLHIV and how these configure so-called 'positive living'. Positive living in this context entails as Benton et al. note,

> disclosing one's HIV-positive status to potential sexual partners, family members, and friends; practicing 'safer sex'; eating well and abstaining from drinking and smoking; and regularly taking medications. More intangibly, positive living, as the name suggests, also requires a marked positive change in attitude and self-perceptions, and demonstrable levels of self-sufficiency, responsibility, and expressed concern about self-care among HIV-positive people.
>
> (Benton et al., 2017:458)

Benton et al. connect this to three ethnographic field sites, Miami, Florida in the US, Chimoio, Mozambique and Freetown, Sierra Leone (Benton et al., 2017:454) and interrogate how temporality functions in the frame of positive living experiences across these sites. I seek to connect their insights with my own focus on neoliberalism and argue that, in the era of 'ending AIDS', health promotions that address PLHIV balance between playing on disciplinary notions of subjection to biomedical adherence, on the one hand, a much more neoliberal notion of security wherein positive living also signifies a return to 'normal' on the other. I seek, in the final analysis, to draw out the three 'categories' (suppression, disclosing and surviving) as part of a discourse where empowerment meets neoliberalism and where discipline meets freedom. In the era of the end of AIDS, what positive living campaigns needs to be critically analyzed, not as a negative analysis of access to and use of ARVs, but rather to tease out what 'problems' such health promotions seek to address, what behaviors they encourage; conversely, how certain behaviors become normative and desirable while others are shunned or discouraged.

Suppress! Disclose! Survive!

If an HIV test is the first step in the treatment cascade for PLHIV, then accessing care and starting on ARVs is the second step. As we have seen, in the age of the end of AIDS, viral load suppression is seen as the successful endpoint for HIV treatment. Epitomized in the 90-90-90 targets, viral suppression has become both the end goal for individual patients as well as communities and indeed nations. This push toward viral suppression has become a hallmark in HIV treatment and prevention initiatives and health care campaigns. Popularized through the concept of 'undetectable', 'becoming undetectable' has become a process of both personal goal setting and in certain instances, a moral obligation (Cormier McSwiggin, 2017; Grace et al., 2015; Persson et al., 2017). In light of evidence showing that undetectable viral loads also ensures that PLHIV cannot transmit HIV onward, the slogan of 'U=U' (undetectable is untransmittable) has emerged as a way of communicating both the science behind ARVs, and as a way of reducing stigma through a focus on the fact that undetectable viral loads makes it impossible to transmit the virus onward even during condomless sex (Eisinger et al., 2019; UNAIDS, 2018; Zamora et al., 2018)

So how is this mediated in health promotions and what comes with such promotions? I want to focus in on perhaps one of the most prolific online HIV health promotions for people living with HIV, the '*HIV Stops with Me*' campaign, and look at how issues of positive living plays on achieving viral suppression yet also is entangled with injunctions to disclose HIV status as well as healthy living advice. Once again, I seek to connect this to both the issues of both temporality that Benton et al. demonstrated in their work but also discipline and personal responsibility. My analysis is not so much a critique of the *HIV Stops with Me* campaign, rather, it is to shed light on how viral load suppression, disclosing HIV status and positive living through healthy habits produce a normative subject that lives with HIV.

The '*HIV Stops with Me*' health promotion was originally developed in New York and is found both online as an HIV resource website and on flyers and billboards that inform people about living with HIV through what the campaigns assert is 'positive talk'. This positive talk is a combination of narratives and testimonies made by people living with HIV and health information produced by medical authorities in terms of what is important to follow once one has become HIV-positive. It is worth noting that the *HIV Stops with Me* health promotion was nominated for 'Best Advertising Campaign' by Gay Lesbian Alliance Against Defamation (GLAAD) and has won a Webby Award for 'Best Health Website'. Other awards include Telly and Davey awards as well as a W3 and the American Graphic Design award.[1] As such, the *HIV Stops with Me* promotion has become somewhat of an icon in terms of the ways in which it empowers PLHIV to tell their own 'positive' stories and offers a way of talking about HIV without stigma.

The *HIV Stops with Me* website contains clickable headings for the following pages: 'video diaries', 'treatment info', 'positive talk', 'event videos', 'resources' and an 'about' section. In the treatment section, for instance, the information that is disseminated follows a narrative wherein the user is met with the statement 'Get on treatment and stay on it. Medication keeps us healthy. Staying undetectable there's effectively no risk of infecting our partners'[2]. The very first message that is being sent to the subject is one which is mediated through a discourse of biomedicalization of health and prevention. Here in the *HIV Stops with Me* campaign, health and responsibility are intimately tied to the consumption of biomedical ART treatment which then both keeps the subject healthy and also keeps 'our' partners from becoming infected. In this narrative, it is the HIV-positive person who is made responsible for both his or her own health as well as making sure that they stay on treatment so that they won't infect others. The *HIV Stops with Me* promotion focuses almost exclusively on the individual and what the individual must do in order to ensure that the subject reaches 'undetectable viral load'. As the health promotion states in regard to the point on 'taking your meds', 'Taking your HIV medications, when and how you are supposed to, is extremely important. This is how you decrease your viral load. If you skip your medication, the virus can take that opportunity to replicate and make more HIV.

By skipping doses, you may develop strains of HIV that are resistant to the medications. Taking the medications gives you control over the virus'.[3] Adherence is highlighted as crucial for PLHIV, and control is rendered possible through adhering to ARVs. Every step of the way the subjectivation process which is taking place is one that highlights a 'you' that is personalized and made singular through the ways in which it is the individual that must adhere, comply and follow a regimented and biomedical script in order to suppress and 'control the virus'. The *HIV Stops with Me* campaign seems to truly be about the 'me' in ending HIV; it is the HIV-positive person that is the final frontier where the virus needs to be contained and suppressed until it reaches undetectable levels.

This is reminiscent of the ways in which Foucault links the investment of education as part and parcel of the neoliberal logic of the 'self' as an entrepreneur; however, here the use of education is educating oneself about one's own HIV status and health. In investing in this sort of knowledge, the *HIV Stops with Me* campaign also implicitly states that educating yourself regarding your own health will pay dividends further down the line. In fact, by investing time and effort in educating themselves, people living with HIV are seen as subjects that need to invest in a broad range of knowledge about their HIV status in an effort to not only stay healthy and live longer but indeed to keep their partners safe and prevent onward transmission of HIV.

This focus on adherence and achieving viral load suppression is, of course, not only found in the *HIV Stops with Me* campaign. One of the clearest examples of the signifying importance accorded to 'becoming undetectable' in the cultural chronicle of the 'end of AIDS' is the emergence of a comic book series aptly titled *The Undetectables*.[4] This comic book directly links to the NYC strategy to 'end the epidemic' through its association with Housing Works, a non-profit organization based in NYC which is 'a healing community of people living with and affected by HIV/AIDS. Our mission is to end the dual crises of homelessness and AIDS through relentless advocacy, the provision of lifesaving services and entrepreneurial businesses that sustain our efforts' (Murphy, 2015). Per *POZ* magazine, Housing Works, in an effort to destigmatize HIV and promote the importance of becoming undetectable as well as adhering to ARVs,

> asked Berlin-based illustrator Rafa Gonzalez to create a comic book about a group of Housing Works superheroes called, *The Undetectables*, who fight shame, stigma and hopelessness in New York's HIV-positive population, empowering folks to get the support they need to take their meds and keep themselves—and their communities—free from AIDS.
>
> (Murphy, 2015)

The Undetectables comic book is part of a larger program run by Housing Works, which focuses on helping community members maintain good health and adhere to ARVs in an effort to reach undetectable levels. As Ginny Shubert, Housing Works senior advisor on research and policy notes,

We felt that we needed to do our part by achieving a community rate of viral load suppression [undetectability] of 80 percent or more [...] We had to figure out how to get our community members to understand the role of taking care of your own health as part of the overall end of the epidemic.

(Murphy, 2015)

The statement from Ginny Shubert recalls the insights from Gagnon and Guta on the importance accorded to community viral load (Gagnon & Guta, 2014; Gagnon & Guta, 2012b; Gagnon & Guta, 2012a) numbers as we have seen earlier in this book. It also highlights, once again, the entanglement between the figure of the community and the figure of the individual in terms of how the end of AIDS is conceptualized through the metric of viral loads. Shubert's statement clearly indicates these entanglements through recourse to the notion that community members have to understand the *individual role* they can play in their own lives, but also as *part of the overall end of the epidemic*. Once again, we see the individualization of the end of AIDS. This is not to say that Housing Works leaves responsibility solely up to the individual. The comic book is only part of the program. Housing Works also provides 'financial incentives as part of a meds-adherence program' (Murphy, 2015). In practice, this entails operating with a three tier program for increasing awareness and motivation for adhering to ARVs, first of which is monetary incentives for testing undetectable every three months. If this does not help in increasing rates of viral suppression, then the system has two more tiers which consist of

a support group where enrollees meet to talk through their adherence issues and derive help from one another. And for the most challenged enrollees – the ones often struggling with mental illness or intermittent or heavy drug use – the program employs directly observed therapy, in which a Housing Works staffer comes to the enrollee's residence daily with meds and watches the enrollee take them.

(Murphy, 2015)

As such, an entire system is in place for the people who need adherence counseling the most, and it is combined with a more holistic approach to adhering to ARVs and thus becoming undetectable. HIV does not end solely with the individual in this case; rather, an entire system of people and care is activated.

Yet, even though this system is remarkable in terms of the care and support being provided, I do want to highlight the signifying role of the comic book strip and the semiotic meaning-making that it provides us with. My critique is not leveled at the Housing Works overall program, far from it. Rather I want to highlight how undetectable has become the new norm within sero identities and that this form of signification might turn out to produce a new normative way for living with HIV, wherein the sole criteria for 'treatment success' and indeed living with HIV is reduced to becoming undetectable.

Heroic suppression

In conceptualizing the very name of *The Undetectables*, Juan Astasio, creative director of Housing Works, notes 'The term '*Undetectables*' just sounded like superheroes to us' (Murphy, 2015). In looking deeper at the comic books, it is easy to see the links between superhero iconography and the message of becoming undetectable. Since space considerations foreclose a close reading of the comic books in their entirety, I want to focus on some of the more obvious aspects of the significance accorded to becoming undetectable.

When first accessing the website for *The Undetectables* online version, the viewer is introduced to a slide show which states, 'you have gotten this far living with HIV. Take the next step with us'. After selecting options for language (English and Spanish), the viewer is introduced to the comic book and its characters. Next up is the home page, where there are four banners to click on: 'find a provider', 'learn the facts', 'read the comic' and 'become a partner'. In the 'learn the facts' section, many of the same issues as we saw in the *HIV Stops with Me* campaign are found. Questions such as 'what is viral load?' and 'what does viral suppression mean?' are included with answers provided by members of *The Undetectables*.

The members of *The Undetectables* are Joyce Green, Spirit Soriano, Virgil Lincoln, Terrence Powers and Tenille Roberts, all of whom have fictional biographies and nicknames, such as 'the relentless advocate' or 'the harm reducer'. Listed after these, are their enemies: Denial, Phear, Apatha, Stigma and Richard Frost, the only human of the villains and a 'right-wing news anchor for the Faux News channel. His conservative agenda masks a sinister plan to rid the world of *The Undetectables* and run the city through anger under his true identity, MALICE'.[5] The fictional bios of these superheroes provide short narratives of when they become HIV-positive and characteristics of the members. We also find them in the 'learn the facts' section of the website. It is here that I want to highlight some of the ways in which 'positive living', as conceptualized by Benton et al., and the entanglements between individual responsibility for one's own health as well as the health of communities (with focus on disclosing HIV status and having a positive outlook on HIV sero status) comes to the fore. I also want to highlight that while these aspects are important and indeed worthwhile to follow up on, they nevertheless might also be read as a form of normative and moralizing enactment of sero status where undetectable becomes normative.

In the 'learn the facts' section, the question is posed, 'what does suppressing my viral load mean for other people?' The answer given is 'Having an undetectable viral load for at least six months and continuing to stay on medication means you are not putting your partner at risk. Consider having an open conversation with your partner or a friend you can trust. Let them know how you're feeling, what you're scared of and how they might be able to help you continue making healthy choices'.[6] The emphasis on not putting *others* at risk is, as we have seen before, part and parcel of the rhetorical framing of the value of becoming undetectable. The value it seems, is not only evaluated in a biomedical sense, but also in a moral sense, if only implicit through the notion that individuals who are undetectable keep others safe. It is interesting to note that throughout my research on the value and framing of 'undetectable=untransmittable' (U=U) and the value of becoming undetectable, very little if anything is accorded to the value this has for intimacy and sex. Undetectable is bracketed as valuable because it keeps PLHIV healthy and/or is framed as making it impossible to transmit HIV onward to others. Yet, the notion that people who become undetectable can find value in having sex without fear of onward transmission is not a focus in any of the health promotions or in the science on becoming undetectable. Sex, even in the age of U=U, is still a 'reluctant object' it seems (Race, 2016). Indeed, sexual pleasure as part of the value of becoming undetectable is never part of the discussion. Rather, undetectable is rendered intelligible only through the notion of 'successful treatment', keeping others 'safe' from HIV and healthy living. Responsibility for one's own health is highlighted in the above and in the *HIV Stops with Me*, as well as responsibility for the health of others. Case in point is the next question on the list.

Here the question is 'how did *The Undetectables* suppress their viral loads?'. The answer given is: 'We found that in our personal experience, taking our medications, getting our viral loads as low as possible and keeping a high level of responsibility over our health has helped us hone and channel our powers, making us even stronger. We became undetectable to prove that we're heroes to ourselves and to the community around us'[7]. Here I argue that we can clearly see the responsibilization of the 'self', a form of biomedical disciplinary regime wherein to become undetectable is to 'keep a high level of responsibility' for one's own health. The valorization of becoming undetectable is clearly linked to the notion that *The Undetectables* are heroes, and thus others who reach undetectable should be considered heroes.

Karen Lloyd has written on *The Undetectables* in terms of it being part of what she calls 'the centering of a new face of HIV' (Lloyd, 2018). Lloyd argues that *The Undetectables*, the subsequent comic and campaign, frame the process of becoming undetectable as something 'cool', 'hip' and heroic, where PLHIV are encouraged to 'change from the inside out' through adhering to and achieving undetectable viral levels (Lloyd, 2018:475). However, Lloyd's argument further states that the comic book series goes beyond promoting awareness, education and promotion of behavior change; rather, *The Undetectables*, and others like it, 're-configure what it means to *be* a person living with HIV in the era of HIV treatment as prevention' (Lloyd, 2018:475). Lloyd focuses particularly on the role of the use of comic or the cartoon imagery as a unique form of mediation (Lloyd, 2018:475). Yet I argue that if we are to take seriously the insights from Paula Treichler (Treichler, 1999) and the work of Kenworthy et al. on the signifying epidemic in an era that proposes that the end of AIDS is near (Kenworthy et al., 2018b; Kenworthy et al., 2018a), then the images and online information are crucial for 'shaping the conditions of possibility for making ourselves up in the image of these characters, assuming perhaps highly affective ways, their behaviors, their values, their aspirations' (Lloyd, 2018:475). I am not here arguing for a naïve form for representational politics wherein people who view and engage with online HIV preventive health promotions blindly follow or are always convinced by the messaging that these health promotions bring to the table. In fact, a lot of research has already been conducted on the function, effectiveness and value of HIV health promotions (Kippax & Van de Ven, 1998; McOwan et al., 2002; Noar et al., 2009). Indeed, one might argue that there is an entire subfield of HIV social science research dedicated to the topic of effective health promotion and communication including media studies, cultural studies, social psychology and sociology of media. My point is not to evaluate if these campaigns work or at what levels they influence actions on part of the people engaging with them. Rather it is to analyze the ways in which HIV campaigns have come to signify what it means to end AIDS, what signifying elements are brought into the conversation and how is responsibility (health, sexual and moral) addressed.

The Detectables? What undetectable can tell us about new norms for HIV status and the notion of viral suppression as success criteria

One might argue that these health promotions, *HIV Stops with Me* and *The Undetectables*, aim at empowering PLHIV to access treatment and partake in a normalization of HIV through both disclosing their HIV status and becoming undetectable, thereby rendering onward HIV transmission impossible. Yet I argue there is a fine balance between empowerment and normalization on the one hand and, on the other hand, normative and moral injunctions to become undetectable. In light of the paradigm of treatment as prevention and the push to get as many people accessing and adhering to ARV treatment, health campaigns such as *HIV Stops with Me* and *The Undetectables* might be linked to what has been called 'pharmaceutical citizenship' (Ecks, 2005). For Ecks, pharmaceutical citizenship is 'the biomedical promise of demarginalization' (Ecks, 2005:241) offered through accessing and consuming different pharmaceuticals for communities often defined by some form of chronic illness such as depression. Variants of this concept have been used in the case of HIV as described in the work of Vinh-Kim Ngyuen and his notion of 'therapeutic citizenship' (Nguyen, 2010). Other variants can be discerned through the concept of 'biosociality' invoked by Paul Rabinow (Rabinow, 1992). Common to these is the focus on how access to citizenship is enacted and redefined by the 'pharmaceuticalization of public health' (Biehl, 2007). A particularly poignant point in our own case here, is one raised by Ecks when he states that not only have pharmacological treatments been framed as a human right, but equally important, is the ways in which pharmacological treatments have been framed as having the ability to restore citizenship by drawing disadvantaged or stigmatized communities back into society (Ecks, 2005:239–241). In the popular press, examples of this type of narrative abound. In a series of articles in *The Guardian* ranging from 2015 to 2019, for instance, there are traces of this sort of being 'drawn back into society'. In an article titled 'HIV and Me', the newspaper covers seven short narratives from across the globe of people living with HIV. Significantly, all of them highlighted how starting treatment was a 'way back' to 'good health', 'love', 'longevity', 'motherhood' and 'acceptance' (Gideon & Gere, 2019). Another piece on the topic of living with HIV from *The Guardian* is called 'Living with HIV: Six Very Different Stories' (Tucker, 2015). In much the same way, accessing ARV treatment and adhering to it is narrated as a way of 'returning to' something: health, acceptance or a form of 'normality'. Others narrate stories of temporality reminiscent of what Benton et al. have described as 'a break' or a 'before and after' diagnosis, a temporality of puncture (Benton et al., 2017).

Becoming undetectable seems to play on a reintegration back into health in the *HIV Stops with Me*, *The Undetectables* and many of the narratives found in popular press and news media outlets. The new norm seems to portray becoming undetectable as both a route to health and a return to normalcy. Yet, as Asha Persson et al. ask: 'in this ambitious environment, what are the implications for citizenship and people's sense of inclusion if they decide to *not* take HIV treatment?' (Persson et al., 2016:362). Alternatively, what are the consequences for those who for whatever reasons fail to achieve viral suppression, or who only achieve this partially and in patchwork intervals of time? In an age where the end of AIDS is heralded as being possible by 2030 and where the end goal of treatment is to achieve undetectable viral load numbers, it seems as though we have reached a new form of 'social contract' for PLHIV. This contract, as it is framed in the aforementioned campaigns, seems to focus on a version of pharmaceutical citizenship wherein there is an 'enjoinment to engage and comply with biomedical solutions on offer in order to fulfill one's obligations as a citizen and become acceptable to society' (Persson et al., 2016:362). It is perhaps a paradox then that, by and large, adhering to and accessing ARV treatment for PLHIV has not only become a way of ensuring health for oneself but almost equally important, to keep others healthy as well. Yet, as we have seen with the controversy around PrEP, not every pharmaceutical drug treatment is met with the same framing. Indeed, if we juxtapose the controversies around PrEP with that of ARV treatment, it seems that while people who adhere to ARVs and achieve viral suppression are framed as literal heroes, those who access PrEP are in certain cases framed as 'Truvada whores'.

Disclosure: positive talk as care of the self

In an earlier chapter of this book, I wrote about how viral load metrics bind the figure of the individual with the figure of the community through the concept of community viral load. This entanglement has, as we have seen, consequences for how HIV health promotions frame the process of becoming undetectable. Returning to *The Undetectables*, we note how the individual person's responsibility for one's own health becomes entangled with the responsibility of keeping others healthy as well. One of the questions in the 'learn the facts' section of *The Undetectables* is 'what does suppressing my viral load do for my community?'. The answer: 'Becoming undetectable is a process with a cascading effect that influences everyone in your community. When you take the first step to seek treatment, you give others the green light to seek treatment for themselves, too. That's what being a hero is all about – being brave enough to take that first step so that you play a critical role in ending the HIV/AIDS epidemic for *every-one*.[8] In a very clear way, this quote shows how the individual's responsibility of becoming undetectable also is part and parcel of a framing that highlights the individual's responsibility to 'take the first step' which then is posited as having a cascading effect on others. On the one hand, there is a clear desire, it seems, to empower and indeed destigmatize HIV. Yet, this very same empowerment seems also to add responsibility to the individual PLHIV. Not only does the person have an individual responsibility to become undetectable for their own sake, there is also the need to take responsibility so that others may follow. Michel Foucault wrote in his later years on the concept of 'the care of the Self' as a mode of caring for oneself through various techniques ranging from dietary to confessional and from corporal to spiritual (Foucault, 2012). For Foucault these techniques were not only forms of caring for the body and the health of the person but also informed ethical and moral care of the self. Foucault states that 'there are different ways to "conduct oneself" morally, different ways for the acting individual to operate, not just as an agent, but as an ethical subject of action'. (Foucault, 2012:26). The point I want to draw out here, in perhaps a very superficial manner is that adherence to ARV, pursuing the endeavor to become undetectable through positive living initiatives such as healthy eating, exercise, disclosing one's HIV status and, in general, obtaining a 'positive' and optimistic outlook on living with HIV can, in many ways, be seen as a form of care of the self. It includes caring for the physical health and wellbeing of the body, but it also involves a conduct that has a form of moral valence, an ethical component that goes beyond, yet is entangled with, the levels of viral suppression. In a way, PLHIV are encouraged to become in many ways 'an ethical subject of action' through positive living programs. Vinh-Kim Nguyen has written something akin to this in his genealogy of HIV counseling in Western Africa (Nguyen, 2013). Nguyen notes that for people newly diagnosed and living with HIV, there lies 'beyond the immediate issue of complying with sexual and pharmaceutical prescriptions, [...] a concern with the care of the self. Underlying counselling is the injunction to "know thyself" in order that appropriate behavior may be achieved. This is ultimately an incitement to make one's self anew' (Nguyen, 2013:S441). In many ways the focus on a care of the self that both focuses on 'knowing thyself' and to 'make one self anew' fits well with what has been previously described as ways that positive living health promotions frame PLHIV as active moral agents that can be empowered through the right techniques of adhering to and living well with HIV. However, this care of the self can only be obtained through collecting information that is in line with bio-medical practices, and in this manner can the subject come to know themselves as 'heroes' living with HIV. The notion that such care of the self for PLHIV is a form of making oneself 'anew' also seems to resonate somewhat with how the 'punctured temporality' before and after diagnosis can be seen as form of 'reintegration' into the social contract of being a pharmaceutical citizen.

The other side of this coin would perhaps be a darker, more conflict-oriented reading wherein this technology of the self is based on a disciplinary regimen meant to contain and individualize responsibility in such a manner that the subject is always already inscribed within an oppressive biomedical matrix of power.

Regardless, I think there is good reason to see these health promotions not only as part of a biopolitical machinery of security and discipline, but perhaps also as prescriptive texts that inform a practice of caring for the self. This might be a normative practice, but nonetheless it does seem to provide a prescriptive way of living with HIV, one that cares for both the body and the soul, so to speak. Vinh-Kim Nguyen addresses something akin to this in terms of HIV counseling and the practice of counseling in general, but he connects specifically HIV counseling to the genealogy of various confessional technologies such as psychoanalysis and the Christian doctrine of confession (Nguyen, 2013). He notes that

> Counselling draws on this heritage but remains much more pragmatic, aiming simply to help clients clarify what they really want and why, hoping to guide them to what's best for them. It is this psychotherapeutic heritage that insists that counsellors not interfere with clients' ultimate desires and that counselling is not telling people what to do.
>
> (Nguyen, 2013:S448)

While I am not here dealing with concealing per se, the traces of the same logic can be discerned in the *HIV Stops with Me*, *The Undetectables* and *It Starts with Me* campaigns. In many ways, they contain the same logic of making sure that PLHIV both comply with adherence to ARVs and disclose HIV status. All of these health promotions promote 'confessing' or disclosing one's sero status and through this process we are told that communal stigma will be reduced and a form of normalcy of HIV status will be achieved.

However, while the health promotions we have looked at so far target the individual with messages of adherence and various other health promoting practices, there is also a clear focus on the responsibility that the individual has toward the community. Whereas the campaigns can be seen as providing prescriptive messaging about adherence and a certain form of care of the self, there is also evidence of what Colvin et al. have called 'caring for the social' (Colvin et al., 2010). Not only is adhering to ARVs and becoming undetectable a form of care of the self, it is also a caring for others through the paradigm of 'treatment as prevention'. Perhaps this is indeed why positive living, as it is now unfolding, can be seen as a form of care of the self; no longer is the ethical and moral imperative to stay healthy centered on the individual self the only focus of HIV treatment. Rather, the ethical imperative to adhere to ARVs is refracted through (1) the communal responsibility to becoming undetectable so as to stop onward transmission of HIV and (2) a moral imperative to reduce communal stigma through disclosing HIV status. Being a responsible pharmaceutical citizen in the age of the end of AIDS seems to signify, as Colvin states, 'both "caring for the self" and/as "caring for the social", whether through forms of political activism, community engagement or simply through contributing to their local cycle of social reproduction' (Colvin et al., 2010:1180) and, might we add here, becoming undetectable thus also untransmittable.

A question to note here briefly is how these forms of health promotions also seem to produce a new normative identity within what we can call 'sero identities'. This new identity seems to be the heroic undetectable subject which might come to displace identities such as HIV-positive as both Karen Lloyd and Adele Clarke et al. ponder (Clarke et al., 2010; Lloyd, 2018). In this chapter titled 'HIV Both Starts and Stops with Me', it is of course also notable that the quote highlights how the individual's responsibility for his/her own health is also bound with 'ending the HIV/AIDS epidemic for *everyone*'.

If, as Deborah Lupton has argued, individual health has become a moral imperative (Lupton, 1995), then to become undetectable seems to produce highly normative and moral imperatives through adhering to ARVs. While I am not disputing that access to and usage of ARVs are a social and personal good, what I am raising is the concern that a new form of 'sero normativity' is emerging wherein individuals who do not reach undetectable levels, who defer from starting treatment right away, or who go on and off treatment for different reasons will be labeled as 'irrational', 'dangerous' or 'failed' subjects. However, as Pound et al.'s literature review shows, there are a myriad of competing rationalities or constraints that are at play when people do not adhere to pharmaceutical treatments, and often times these people have both understandable and logical reasons for not taking their medicines (Pound et al., 2005). The focus on undetectability has also become a focal point for community and activist critiques.

The Detectables?

Tamas Bereczky, working for the European Patients' Academy, penned in the BMJ an essay titled, 'U=U is a blessing: but only for patients with access to HIV treatment' (Bereczky, 2019). In the essay Tamas, an openly HIV-positive man since 2003 (Bereczky, 2019), argues that while U=U has been a tremendous boon for the many people who live with HIV, it has also set into motion new norms and ethical dilemmas. First of all, Bereczky highlights that the U=U movement only works for the people who have access to treatment, and that the enormous focus on becoming undetectable might indeed obscure the fact that a great many people still lack access to ARVs. Cases mentioned are Serbia, which has stopped conducting viral load testing since 2017, and Russia, where only 42 percent of all PLHIV are on treatment (Bereczky, 2019). This is compounded by the fact that even people on treatment might be on and off treatment due to drug stockouts, as demonstrated by a 2018 study in Central and Eastern Europe which showed that nine out of 23 countries had reported stock-outs of ARV (Gokengin et al., 2018). This shows that becoming a hero as in *The Undetectables* is reliant upon so much more than individual agency and will to become undetectable. Structural issues, such as access to ARVs, drug stockouts and medical system navigation, all influence how and when people achieve or don't achieve undetectable levels. Bereczky's argument focuses upon access to ARVs and structural issues, such as stockouts anti-LGBTQI laws and state-sanctioned homophobia such as that in Russia, Hungary and Poland (Bereczky, 2019). His solution is to increase access to ARVs and develop smaller, more affordable viral load tests in an effort to ensure that all PLHIV have access to these technologies.

However, we can also trace another form of critique against the iconography and discourse found in *The Undetectables*, perhaps best understood as a critique of norms and normativity. An example of this comes from an article published on the website of *The BodyPro* which is dedicated to delivering news, science and medical information on HIV to people living with HIV and clinicians.

The article, 'We need to talk about the downside of U=U' was penned by George Johnson (Johnson, 2020), an openly HIV-positive man who works as a community health care worker and activist. In a biting critique of U=U, Johnson provides us with an important corrective or supplement to, the U=U discourse and the notion that the end of AIDS will, and can only, come about if people who live with HIV reach undetectable levels of HIV.

Johnson states that he at first was 'all for' the U=U slogan, but that he now, three years later, feels different. He notes that using U=U as a framework for reducing stigma

> has become nothing more than a gesture to prove that the bodies of people living with HIV are safe to have sex with, and I believe it has added another layer of oppression to Black people's plight in the HIV epidemic.
>
> (Johnson, 2020)

His rationale for reaching this conclusion comes from providing us with a mediation on the entanglements between access to ARVs, normativity for what it means to live with HIV in the age of U=U and what we mean by 'healthy' when one lives with HIV. His first critique is that the U=U movement seems to forget and leave out the many vulnerable and most affected by HIV; that is, the U=U centers viral suppression as a marker of health above and beyond anything else, yet discussions about barriers to access are often omitted in these conversations.

Secondly, Johnson states that while the science behind U=U is indeed groundbreaking and important, as well as being recommended by all medical guidelines and strategies, it fails to recognize that undetectable does not equal healthy nor is it a status that, once attained, is always manageable (Johnson, 2020). Once again, Johnson's remark highlights the, at times, difficult and uneven road to becoming undetectable. Perhaps more important in the context of U=U and the cartoon of *The Undetectables* is the critique of undetectable as the *sole* goal of PLHIV. Johnson rightly highlights the fact that becoming undetectable is not always the same as being healthy. In fact, a doxic focus on U=U might obscure focus on how notions of health are conceptualized when it comes to people who are living with HIV. Indeed, Johnson's comments on the overt focus on reaching undetectable levels, as the sole criteria for PLHIV in terms of health, resonate with several public health researchers who state that the 90-90-90 targets' overt focus on viral suppression should be supplemented by other aspects of human health and indeed argue for a move 'beyond the 90-90-90 targets'. In comparing the message of the undetectable and the work of health promotions such as *HIV Stops with Me*, its easy to see the tensions and norms taking shape.

On the one hand, few would argue that U=U is not scientific, or that its not a vital part of the effort to end AIDS. However, on the other hand, the introduction of U=U and the focus on viral suppression has also created a new set of binaries that in turn have ethical, social and political ramifications.

Returning to Johnson's critique of U=U, he also draws our attention to a few other aspects of the U=U slogan that are worth quoting here while we also keep in mind the message of *The Undetectables*.

Acknowledging that U=U is an important part of the toolbox in HIV efforts, Johnson nevertheless also notes what he takes to be an important downside to U=U: rather than only being a tool for empowerment as highlighted by *The Undetectables*, Johnson states that becoming undetectable has in certain cases been a way to weaponize HIV status and thus create a hierarchy within HIV affected communities (Johnson, 2020). He illustrates this by way of an Instagram account that was called 'TheUndetectableList', which has since been taken down by Instagram. The account was dedicated to exposing people who were HIV-positive but not undetectable. In so doing, Johnson highlights how moral and ethical issues arise and how people who are HIV-positive but not detectable are placed in precarious and even dangerous situations exemplified by the Instagram case. I want to highlight one last aspect of Johnson's article and critique of the downside of U=U before I connect his critique to *The Undetectables*.

One of my arguments in this chapter has been to highlight some of the complexities that the push for viral load suppression has created on the road to ending AIDS. Since viral load suppression has become both the goal of individual HIV treatment as well as a metric used for monitoring the progress toward the end of AIDS on a communal level, undetectability has become the new norm. This norm is one that is both individualized, as we can see in the critique provided by Johnson, and massified through the monitoring of communal viral load metrics. Perhaps, bluntly put, what counts as successful HIV treatment and the new norm for such success seems to be achieving detectability on all scales.

For Johnson, this also has ramifications for *who* is responsible for the end of AIDS. Johnson states that

> HIV-positive people cannot be responsible for the burden of the work in ending the epidemic. We are often placed in positions where we carry the responsibility and accountability for the sexual health of others. Our 'undetectable' status also shouldn't be used as a badge of honor to tell people it is 'safe to sleep with us' or interact with us without fear of contracting the virus.
>
> (Johnston, 2020)

Johnson's critique of the dogmatic focus of U=U and its normative and ethical fallout goes straight to the heart of my argument in this chapter: it shows us how responsibility is placed on PLHIV in terms of their own health but, more importantly, the health of others.

HIV Stops with Me and *The Undetectables* play on tropes such as empowerment, heroism and personal choice in connection to becoming undetectable and thus also doing 'your part' in ending the epidemic. Johnson, however, alerts us to the fact that if viral load suppression becomes the sole focus and sole success criteria for HIV treatment, then we risk losing sight of a more holistic approach to the HIV epidemic and what it can mean to live with HIV in the age of the end of AIDS. Drawing our attention to these complexities does not mean that we need or should disown slogans such as U=U or cast doubt on the impact of viral load suppression. Rather, it entails showing how new norms for sexual responsibility and accountability have emerged through the focus on undetectability. Becoming undetectable signifies, in this new matrix, heroism, personal responsibility, personal achievement, making sure that one practices safe sex and commits to ending AIDS, we are told, through campaigns such as *HIV Stops with Me* and *The Undetectables*. My analysis here is not an indictment of these campaigns; they clearly have their place in the overall strategy to limit onward HIV transmission, combat stigma and ensure people who live with HIV are seen, heard and receive the treatment they both deserve and need.

However, the downside of U=U is the lack of focus on the obstacles that might arise on the road to becoming undetectable. It also fails to acknowledge the many reasons people might not start right away on ARVs or why they might discontinue using ARVs.

Here, concerns range from side effects, treatment effectiveness, doubts about the need to start treatment right away, feelings of health and wellbeing, a reluctance to commit to daily regimens as well as structural issues such as housing, unemployment and stigma (Amico et al., 2007; Fagan et al., 2010; Gwadz et al., 2015; Walsh et al., 2001). To be fair, the Housing Works project, which spawned *The Undetectables*, *does* account for many of these aspects in their work. As such, it is less Housing Works that I am here analyzing, but, more so, the ways in which undetectability as a norm and as a moral imperative that makes the individual both responsible for their own health and that of others that I am here critiquing. Housing Works as an organization *does* offer a holistic program and focuses on issues of stigma, mental health, drug use and homelessness. Yet *The Undetectables*, even though well-intended, play on many of the same tropes that large organizations such as UNAIDS and PEPFAR do: that is, the ultimate goal of HIV treatment is viral load suppression, both at the individual level and at the level of the population.

Yet, accounts like Johnson's and Bereczky's problematize the ways in which undetectable is the 'be-all and end-all' goal of HIV strategies. On a more theoretical level, it also alerts us to the ways in which undetectability as a 'solution' suddenly also becomes its own problem space. It sets into motion new ethical dilemmas as well as normative notions of responsibility and accountability and thus becomes its own form of problem – even if it has been lauded as part of the 'solution' to the problem of HIV.

The danger, as I have argued in this chapter, is that undetectability becomes so doxic that we are left with no other measurement for what can constitute successful positive living with HIV. Furthermore, the overt focus on U=U might displace attention away from those who do not become undetectable as well as other health needs for people living with HIV.

Finally, as exemplified through the Instagram account 'TheUndetectableList', drawn to its logical conclusion, people living with HIV but who do not reach undetectable might end up being cast not as heroes, but indeed as villains.

Concluding remarks

As Beckmann has noted, many of the aforementioned mechanisms in the global drive to end AIDS has shifted the burden of responsibility for the success of heavily funded programs onto the shoulders of the patient and promotes a concept of life whose value is predominantly biological (Beckmann, 2013). In such an optic of what it will mean to end AIDS, people who do not adhere, fail to reach viral suppression or go on and off ARVs are not only in danger of not being 'heroes' but might indeed become further marginalized on the road to the SDG goal of ending AIDS by 2030. Indeed, as Persson et al. argues, this new shift in HIV treatment and prevention regimes might end up creating new marginalities wherein those who are 'detectable' become stigmatized, thus becoming 'marginalized pharmaceutical citizens' (Persson et al., 2016). There is another layer to this which is historically significant and which is of interests here. Since the beginning of the HIV/AIDS epidemic, there has been an immense battle conducted by activists, patients, doctors and NGOs to establish HIV treatment as a human right (Epstein, 1996; Gruskin & Tarantola, 2008). Gruskin and Tarantola note that great strides have been made in at least acknowledging and incorporating parts of human rights frameworks in terms of access to treatment and prevention regimes globally, at least in national action plans and strategies (Gruskin & Tarantola, 2008:s130). However, they also note that the real utilization and practical applications as well as the outcomes of these plans have not been sufficiently explored (Gruskin & Tarantola, 2008:S130). I am in agreement with them in that the battle for human rights and the right to HIV drug treatments is still far from over. However, and here I quote Asha Persson et al., there are

> growing concerns among some activists and researchers that the rush to end the epidemic will override hard-won human rights and justice-based responses to HIV championed by affected communities in Australia and elsewhere by putting increasing moral pressure on people to do their duty and act responsibly for the greater good, thereby undermining their right to autonomy, dignity and freedom from discrimination.
>
> (Persson et al., 2016:372)

The *It Starts with Me* (England), the *HIV Stops with Me* (US) and *The Undetectables* (NYC) health promotions all seek to empower PLHIV and ensure that PLHIV are healthy and not the subjects of stigma and discrimination. None of these health campaigns are ill-intended nor malign, far from it. They represent, to an extent, initiatives wherein PLHIV and organizations come together and work toward a common goal of providing information on treatment, care and how we all can contribute to the end of AIDS.

Yet, the focus on biomedical solutions and suppression of viral loads as being the sole success criteria for successful treatment belies the many complex and entangled issues that need to be tackled if the promise to end AIDS, made in the UN *Sustainable Development Goals* and in the *Political Declaration on the End of AIDS* is to come true (Sidibé et al., 2016). It seems that there is a fine line between empowerment and obligation, between rights and pressures and between suppression of viral loads and suppression of those people who cannot achieve suppressed viral loads. The homogenizing tendencies in focusing only on viral load suppression as the end of AIDS might, in the end, come to create a form of pharmaceutical citizenship which can become divisive by working to define *new margins* of inclusion and exclusion (Persson et al., 2016:372). Who is acting 'wisely' and who is not in the eyes of biomedicine, who is acting responsibly and who is not, who is defined as a proper HIV citizen and who will be relegated to the categories of 'difficult patients', 'irrational', 'Truvada whores' or 'chem sex users'? These are all questions that arise in the entanglements between the ways in which pharmaceuticals have enabled PLHIV to live long lives *with* HIV instead of dying *from* HIV. At the same time, since treatment is no longer just treatment but also prevention, becoming undetectable is no longer just a personal process or road to being healthy: it has become part and parcel of international and national health care strategies aimed at ending the HIV/AIDS epidemic. Put bluntly, becoming undetectable is no longer only a personal goal or a personal virtue: it has become instrumentalized as a form of public health strategy.

I titled the prior chapter, *HIV both starts and stops with me* as a pun on the English health promotion campaign *It Starts with Me* and *HIV Stops with Me* in the US. While the pun itself might not be very unique, I do want to draw out some implications for the end of AIDS as it is proposed within the current HIV efforts. First of all, to end AIDS as it is framed in these health promotions indicates a strong push toward both HIV testing, but also on adhering to ARVs and ultimately becoming undetectable. In all of the health promotions, there is a strong underlying premise that becoming undetectable has several effects, many of them beyond the suppression of viral loads. Ending AIDS is not only framed as a personal responsibility, or rather, HIV starts and stops with the individual through becoming undetectable. In the era of treatment as prevention, responsibility for PLHIV in 'doing their part' is not only taking care of themselves, but rather, through the care that they do toward obtaining a suppressed viral load and living healthily, they are also framed as taking responsibility for others.

Secondly, the shift that ARVs have ushered in also signifies a new era of HIV subjectivities. Going from the early 'healthy selves' (HIV-negative) and the 'diseased others' (the AIDS patient) (Lloyd, 2018:481) to 'undetectable' and 'detectable' has produced new forms of living with HIV. It also has meant as we see in the above health promotions a new set of binaries and new forms of moral and ethical prescriptions. I am in agreement with Lloyd when she writes that

> these novel modes of subjectification may be generative of a re-drawing of moral boundaries between those who can and do make themselves up as undetectable, who are disciplined enough to protect their own health and that of their communities through these practices of pharmaceutical and virological self-governance, and those who are not, who cannot be 'an Undetectable', particularly those that lack access to care and/or treatment, or whose multi-drug resistance make it difficult for them to sustain long term viral suppression.
>
> (Lloyd, 2018:481)

New moral boundaries are indeed being drawn if we look at the scholarship that has emerged in the wake of treatment as prevention. Several studies do indeed support this claim (Bernays, Paparini, Seeley & Rhodes, 2017; Cormier McSwiggin, 2017; Persson, 2013, 2016; Persson, Newman & Ellard, 2017; Persson et al., 2016; Sandset, 2019). Connecting this to the title of this chapter, perhaps there is good cause to say that within the era of the end of AIDS, biomedicalization has meant that responsibility has been shifted onto the individual living with HIV as both the site of containment of the virus, but also as the locus of continual vigilance against failing to adhere. The beginning of the end of AIDS in these health promotions seems to start with the HIV test and end with the pursuit of a suppressed viral load. Between these two lies an incitement to discourse, or rather an incitement to disclose portrayed as a way of taking moral responsibility of ending HIV stigma. While all of this can be, and indeed probably is, empowering in certain cases and at certain times, my argument has been that we need to be careful in framing the end of AIDS in terms that will displace rights with obligations, replace community with individual and make structural drivers invisible while highlighting individual and biomedical solutions to an epidemic that we know, all too well, is driven by social inequality.

Notes

1　See the *HIV Stops with Me* About page; http://hivstopswithme.org/about/
2　See the *HIV Stops with Me* Home page; http://hivstopswithme.org/
3　See the *HIV Stops with Me* Treatment Info page; http://hivstopswithme.org/treatment-info/
4　See the *The Undetectables* comic book webpage; https://liveundetectable.org/comics
5　See the list of characters; https://liveundetectable.org/comics
6　See the Learn the Facts webpage; https://liveundetectable.org/learn
7　See the Learn the Facts webpage; https://liveundetectable.org/learn
8　See the Learn the Facts webpage; https://liveundetectable.org/learn, original italics in the quote

References

Amico, K. R., Konkle-Parker, D., Cornman, D., Barta, W., Ferrer, R., Norton, W., ... Fisher, W. (2007). Reasons for ART non-adherence in the Deep South: Adherence needs of a sample of HIV-positive patients in Mississippi. *AIDS Care, 19*(10), 1210–1218.

Beckmann, N. (2013). Responding to medical crises: AIDS treatment, responsibilisation and the logic of choice. *Anthropology and Medicine, 20*(2), 160–174.

Benton, A., Sangaramoorthy, T., & Kalofonos, I. (2017). Temporality and positive living in the age of HIV/AIDS--A multi-sited ethnography. *Current Anthropology, 58*(4), 454.

Bereczky, T. (2019). U= U is a blessing: But only for patients with access to HIV treatment: An essay by Tamás Bereczky. *BMJ, 366*, l5554.

Bernays, S., Paparini, S., Seeley, J., & Rhodes, T. (2017). "Not taking it will just be like a sin": Young people living with HIV and the stigmatization of less-than-perfect adherence to antiretroviral therapy. *Medical anthropology, 36*(5), 485–499.

Biehl, J. G., & Eskerod, T. (2007). *Will to live: AIDS therapies and the politics of survival.* Princeton, NJ: Princeton University Press.

Clarke, A. E., Shim, J. K., Mamo, L., Fosket, J. R., & Fishman, J. R. (2010). Biomedicalization: Technoscientific transformations of health, illness, and US biomedicine. *Biomedicalization: Technoscience, Health, and Illness in the US, 68*(2):47–87.

Colvin, C. J., Robins, S., & Leavens, J. (2010). Grounding 'responsibilisation talk': Masculinities, citizenship and HIV in Cape Town, South Africa. *The Journal of Development Studies, 46*(7), 1179–1195.

Cormier Mcswiggin, C. (2017). Moral adherence: HIV treatment, undetectability, and stigmatized viral loads among Haitians in South Florida. *Medical Anthropology, 36*(8), 714–728.

Ecks, S. (2005). Pharmaceutical citizenship: Antidepressant marketing and the promise of demarginalization in India. *Anthropology and Medicine, 12*(3), 239–254.

Eisinger, R. W., Dieffenbach, C. W., & Fauci, A. S. (2019). HIV viral load and transmissibility of HIV infection: Undetectable equals untransmittable. *JAMA, 321*(5), 451–452.

Epstein, S. (1996). *Impure science: AIDS, activism, and the politics of knowledge.* Berkeley, CA: University of California Press.

Fagan, J. L., Bertolli, J., & McNaghten, A. D. (2010). Understanding people who have never received HIV medical care: a population-based approach. *Public Health Reports, 125*(4), 520–527.

Foucault, Michel. (2012). *Discipline and punish: The birth of the prison.* New York, NY: Vintage.

Gagnon, M., & Guta, A. (2012a). Mapping community viral load and social boundaries: Geographies of stigma and exclusion. *AIDS, 26*(12), 1577–1578.

Gagnon, M., & Guta, A. (2012b). Mapping HIV community viral load: Space, power and the government of bodies. *Critical Public Health, 22*(4), 471–483.

Gagnon, M., & Guta, A. (2014). HIV viral load: A concept analysis and critique. *Research and Theory for Nursing Practice, 28*(3), 204–227.

Gokengin, D., Oprea, C., Begovac, J., Horban, A., Zeka, A. N., Sedlacek, D. ... Banhegyi, D. (2018). HIV care in Central and Eastern Europe: How close are we to the target? *International Journal of Infectious Diseases, 70*, 121–130.

Grace, D., Chown, S. A., Kwag, M., Steinberg, M., Lim, E., & Gilbert, M. (2015). Becoming 'undetectable': Longitudinal narratives of gay men's sex lives after a recent HIV diagnosis. *AIDS Education and Prevention, 27*(4), 333–349.

Gruskin, S., & Tarantola, D. (2008). Universal access to Hiv prevention, treatment and care: Assessing the inclusion of human rights in international and national strategic plans. *AIDS (London, England)*, *22*(Suppl. 2), S123.

Gwadz, M., Cleland, C. M., Applegate, E., Belkin, M., Gandhi, M., Salomon, N. … Wolfe, H. (2015). Behavioral intervention improves treatment outcomes among HIV-infected individuals who have delayed, declined, or discontinued antiretroviral therapy: A randomized controlled trial of a novel intervention. *AIDS and Behavior*, *19*(10), 1801–1817.

Johnson, George (2020). We need to talk about the downside of U=U, *The BodyPro*. Retrieved from https://www.thebody.com/article/downside-u-equals-u.

Kenworthy, N., Thomann, M., & Parker, R. (2018a). Critical perspectives on the 'end of Aids'. *Global Public Health*, *13*(8), 1–3.

Kenworthy, N., Thomann, M., & Parker, R. (2018b). From a global crisis to the 'end of AIDS': New epidemics of signification. *Global Public Health*, *13*(8), 960–971.

Kippax, S., & Van De Ven, P. (1998). An epidemic of orthodoxy? Design and methodology in the evaluation of the effectiveness of HIV health promotion. *Critical Public Health*, *8*(4), 371–386.

Lloyd, K. C. (2018). Centring 'being undetectable' as the new face of HIV: Transforming subjectivities via the discursive practices of HIV treatment as prevention. *BioSocieties*, *13*(2), 470–493.

Lupton, D. (1995). *The imperative of health: Public health and the regulated body*. London: Sage.

Mcowan, A., Gilleece, Y., Chislett, L., & Mandalia, S. (2002). Can targeted HIV testing campaigns alter health-seeking behaviour? *AIDS Care*, *14*(3), 385–390.

Mendel, Gideon, & Gere, David (2019). HIV and me: 'I decided to fight: I always wanted the body of a wrestler'. *The Guardian*. Retrieved from https://www.theguardian.com/society/2019/nov/09/hiv-across-the-world-selfies-and-stories-10-year-project-gideon-mendel.

Murphy, Tim (2015). Suppression superheroes. POZ M*agazine*. Retrieved from https://www.poz.com/article/suppression-superheroes-27628-3266.

Nguyen, V.-K. (2010). *The republic of therapy: Triage and sovereignty in West Africa's time of AIDS*. Durham: Duke University Press.

Nguyen, V.-K. (2013). Counselling against HIV in Africa: A genealogy of confessional technologies. *Culture, Health and Sexuality*, *15*(Suppl. 4), S440–S452.

Noar, S. M., Palmgreen, P., Chabot, M., Dobransky, N., & Zimmerman, R. S. (2009). A 10-year systematic review of HIV/AIDS mass communication campaigns: Have we made progress? *Journal of Health Communication*, *14*(1), 15–42.

Persson, A. (2013). Non/infectious corporealities: tensions in the biomedical era of 'HIV normalisation'. *Sociology of Health & Illness*, *35*(7), 1065–1079.

Persson, A. (2016). 'The world has changed': Pharmaceutical citizenship and the reimagining of serodiscordant sexuality among couples with mixed HIV status in Australia. *Sociology of Health & Illness*, *38*(3), 380–395.

Persson, A., Newman, C. E., & Ellard, J. (2017). Breaking binaries? Biomedicine and serostatus borderlands among couples with mixed HIV status. *Medical Anthropology*, *36*(8), 699–713.

Persson, A., Newman, C. E., Mao, L., & De Wit, J. (2016). On the margins of pharmaceutical citizenship: Not taking HIV medication in the 'treatment revolution' era. *Medical Anthropology Quarterly*, *30*(3), 359–377.

Pound, P., Britten, N., Morgan, M., Yardley, L., Pope, C., Daker-White, G., & Campbell, R. (2005). Resisting medicines: A synthesis of qualitative studies of medicine taking. *Social Science and Medicine, 61*(1), 133–155.

Rabinow, P. (1992). *Artificiality and enlightenment: From sociobiology to biosociality.* In: *Essays on the Anthropology of Reason.* Princeton, NJ: Princeton University Press.

Race, K. (2016). Reluctant objects: Sexual pleasure as a problem for HIV biomedical prevention. *GLQ: a Journal of Lesbian and Gay Studies, 22*(1), 1–31.

Sandset, T. (2019). 'HIV both starts and stops with me': Configuring the neoliberal sexual actor in HIV prevention. *Sexuality & Culture, 23*(2), 657–673.

Sidibé, M., Loures, L., & Samb, B. (2016). The UNAIDS 90–90–90 target: A clear choice for ending AIDS and for sustainable health and development. *Journal of the International AIDS Society, 19*(1), 21133.

Treichler, P. A. (1999). *How to have theory in an epidemic: Cultural chronicles of AIDS.* Durham: Duke University Press.

Tucker, Eleanor (2015). Living with HIV: Six very different stories. *The Guardian.* Retrieved from https://www.theguardian.com/society/2015/mar/22/living-with-hiv-30 -years-on.

UNAIDS. (2018). *Undetectable= Untransmittable. Public health and HIV Viral Load Suppression.* Geneva: UNAIDS.

Walsh, J. C., Horne, R., Dalton, M., Burgess, A., & Gazzard, B. (2001). Reasons for non-adherence to antiretroviral therapy: Patients' perspectives provide evidence of multiple causes. *AIDS Care, 13*(6), 709–720.

Zamora, J., Precht, A., Catrambone, J., & Adeyemi, O. (2018). *Undetectable= untransmittable: Transforming perceptions around HIV prevention and transmission.* Conference proceeding. Retrieved from https://apha.confex.com/apha/2019/meetin gapi.cgi/Paper/443007?filename=2019_Abstract443007.html&template=Word.

8 Conclusion

A tentative end to AIDS?

Ending. An end or final part of something. End. A final part of something, especially a period of time, an activity, or a story. A goal or desired result. Eventually, come to a specified place or situation. A person's death.

– Oxford Online Dictionary

I have tried in this book to reflect on the notion of ending AIDS, what it has entailed in the science of HIV and how it has come to be represented. At the heart of this lies a specific focus on 'targeted' interventions that is concerned either with space or with 'key populations'. In following the traces of the end of AIDS, I have argued that the end of AIDS is also a form of a signifying epidemic as coined by Paula Trechiler (Treichler, 1999) and later followed up in the work of Kenworthy et al. (Kenworthy, Thomann, & Parker, 2018). In arguing for this perspective, I have mapped some of the intersecting pathways that lead to the consolidation of the slogan 'end of AIDS'. Among these have been the focus on epidemiological modeling which laid some of the groundwork for the push for a narrative that fronted the end of AIDS. This, in combination with novel biomedical treatment regimes, has, as I have argued, become a cornerstone of the global HIV effort. Finally, with the backdrop of fiscal austerity and the financial crisis, targeted programs and interventions have become the name of the game to maximize impact.

However, my primary argument has been that the end of AIDS as we see it today cannot be reduced to its biomedical, technological and economic parts. Rather, I have tried to argue that these inform and are in turn informed by the semiotic economy in which they are inserted. Each of the chapters has tried to map one part of the end of AIDS narrative, be that mapping, molecular tracing or health promotion campaigns and the rollout of PrEP.

Concluding on the end of AIDS is an impossible task not only because the 2030 deadline pushed by the UN SDGs is still 10 years out, but more so because it is not altogether clear what the end of AIDS actually will entail. If we are to draw out some lessons from the pages in this book, I think I want to conclude with a few observations on what the end of AIDS signifies and what it doesn't seem to signify.

If we use the initial definition of what 'ending' means (provided by the OED), then we can perhaps also tease these issues out. Firstly, the ending seems to imply 'the final part of something, a period of time, an activity or a story'. This highlights the connection that the end of AIDS narrative has to it a certain kind of periodization. Indeed, the notion that we are currently living in the 'end days of AIDS' or a 'post-AIDS' era has been analyzed by several scholars (Ledin & Benjamin, 2019; Lewis et al., 2015; Rofes, 2015). However, what does such an end or post-AIDS narrative bespeak? On the surface of it, it signals an end to AIDS-related deaths as in the former UNAIDS strategy *Getting to Zero*, where the slogan was 'zero new infections, zero AIDS-related deaths and zero discrimination' (UNAIDS, 2010). It also might be connected to the fact that with ARV treatment, HIV is now seen more as a lifelong chronic disease that you live with and do not die from. Thurka Sangramoorthy has written well on the topic of chronicity and the end of AIDS (Sangaramoorthy, 2018). HIV as a chronic condition and its connection to a post-AIDS temporality seems to signify HIV as a crisis of the past while signaling its current status as a chronic condition maintained through adherence to biomedical treatment (Sangaramoorthy, 2018:992). However, as Sangaramoorthy underscores the hope signaled by the 'end of AIDS' and post-AIDS rhetoric and its emphasis of HIV as a chronic condition 'obscures the sense of protracted uncertainty and precarious life conditions experienced by those who have lived and continue to live in the shadows of the epidemic – including poor women, people of color and transgender individuals' (Sangaramoorthy, 2018:992). If the end of AIDS is heralded as the end of HIV as a crisis, then Sangaramoorthy's insights remind us of the countless people who do not have access to treatment, stable health services and who are in and out of care due to the precariousness of their life situations. I have tried to think problematically around these issues concerning the 90-90-90 targets as well as concerning what 'undetectable' signifies in the many health promotions that are playing on the heroism and individual responsibility of becoming undetectable. I have also tried to make the case that this also is found in PrEP campaigns where personal responsibility, market choice and rational risk calculation come to intersect with pleasure, desire and sex.

The end of AIDS as a historical period mostly manifested in the notion of a post-AIDS period or a post-crisis time seems to belie the fact that many people still labor under conditions that are far from conducive to an end to AIDS. The hopeful conceptualization of an end to AIDS and post-AIDS era is undermined by

> crumbling health systems, and rising social, economic and political inequalities which give way to a pervasive sense of uncertainty that makes HIV less a 'break' from temporally 'normal' lives than an unexceptional and a common experience in many contexts. These multiple temporal experiences of HIV make for an uncertain and unpredictable future not necessarily bound to the present or past.
>
> (Sangaramoorthy, 2018)

The multiple temporalities of the end of AIDS are worth following up on here in the concluding chapter. I started out stating that I sought to problematize what the end of AIDS signifies, and it seems clear here at the end that one such signifying problematic is the issue of what it can mean in a temporal sense.

The end of AIDS envisioned through the 90-90-90 targets has many potential pitfalls, some of which I have mapped in previous chapters. However, one aspect that is relevant for the notion of temporality is how these 90-90-90 targets profess to offer a neutral and objective set of metrics that can track progress toward 'the end of AIDS'. However, it also produces what I have called earlier, its 'non-synchronous others', that is, the 10-10-10. These communities are oftentimes left outside of the discourse of what it will mean to end AIDS, and this highlights Sangaramoorthy's notion of the multiplicities of temporal experiences within a post-AIDS era. If, in some ways, the end of AIDS and post-AIDS narratives have been shaped by the turn from fatal to chronic in terms of what it means to live with HIV and not die from AIDS, then Sangaramoorthy urges us to shift our perspectives onto chronicity as a concept to better understand the end of AIDS narrative. The U=U campaign, *The Undetectables*, as well as *HIV Stops with Me* and other campaigns mentioned in this book all focus on the turn from fatal to chronic and indeed a return to normalcy for people living with HIV. As such, chronicity and the end of AIDS can be read as a way of also reducing stigma as we have seen, moving the language away from 'death sentence' and 'fatal disease' (Dilmitis et al., 2012). These linguistic shifts speak toward how even at the end of AIDS, HIV is still a signifying epidemic, one that continually is producing new linguistic meanings at the intersection of the social, biomedical and technical. This turn toward chronicity and of 'living with HIV' rather than dying from it, clearly embeds the end of AIDS in the temporality of biomedicine and its notions of time (Baum et al., 2010). Chronicity and chronic disease are understood as encompassing persistent symptoms over a longer temporal course, often understood as over an entire life course, oftentimes also with varying degrees of intensities as well as no curative treatment. In the shift from fatal to chronic and from crisis to post-AIDS and the end of AIDS, there has been a shift, Sangaramoorthy argues, from 'acute' to 'chronic' that postulates a natural evolving and, oftentimes, inevitable medical reality for PLHIV, yet this obscures HIV chronicity as induced by bio-technological advances and its entanglements with ongoing crisis within affected communities (Sangaramoorthy, 2018:984).

As such, in the case of HIV, the sense of chronicity is entangled with continual ARV adherence and treatment thus the chronicity of HIV is contingent upon also a life long course of being intimately connected to both ARVs and health care systems. This is part of why the turn to chronicity in the discourse of post-AIDS narratives can obfuscate some of the potential pitfalls of living with HIV even in a post-AIDS era. Due to HIV as a chronic disease and its reliance upon ARVs, people in precarious health care systems or due to discrimination, criminalization or other systemic drivers, might fall in and out of care and thus also adherence to ARVs. Case in point is the housing crisis in many of the large urban centers in the US such as New York, Los Angeles and San Francisco – a fact that has been noted recently (Tung and Jungwirth, 2017). For Sangaramoothy, this leads to the conclusion that HIV chronicity, in the age of the end of AIDS, signifies not inevitable progress toward the end of AIDS, nor even a post-crisis moment within the HIV epidemic. Rather, she contends that

> HIV is a chronic crisis in the US South as in many other regions of the world signaling disparate HIV infection and treatment rates among the poor and socially marginalized. HIV chronicity, then, does very little to substantiate the logic of the 'end of AIDS'; rather it reinforces the unending possibility of suffering, poverty, and illness.
>
> (Sangaramoorthy, 2018:985)

This reorientation is important to keep in mind as it shifts chronicity from a bio-medical understanding of success to a more problematizing inquiry into what post-AIDS chronicity can mean at the end of AIDS. If HIV chronicity can be understood as also the experience of crisis as a constant as Vigh has stated (Vigh, 2008:10), then chronicity shifts our understanding of the end of AIDS as an event or interruption to 'a state of constant precarity. It brings into view what the "end of AIDS" obscures' as Sangaramoorthy states (Sangaramoorthy, 2018:992). I have tried in this book to problematize the end of AIDS along similar lines. By inquiring what new norms, forms of surveillance as well as new forms of signification, emerge in the discourse of the end of AIDS, I have also sought to unpack some of the hidden and potential pitfalls of this end. As such, the end of AIDS in this optic does not signal an ending per se, rather it signals the continual generation of new configurations of norms, sexual citizenships, fields of power and notions of risk, responsibility but also pleasure and desire. In such an optic, it makes little sense of talking about an 'end to AIDS'.

The 'post' in post-AIDS and the 'end' in ending AIDS

One of the most vexing questions in postcolonial studies has been 'what is the post in postcolonial?'. For some, it has signaled a time period that is after colonialism. However, for most, it has signaled a form of epistemological foundation for understanding both the impact of colonialism and imperialism but also as a form of critique and investigating the 'specter of colonialism' (Bhabha, 2012; Fanon, 2008; Loomba, 2007; Said, 2003; Spivak, 1999). Without going into detail about the discussion on the post in postcolonialism, I want to briefly reflect on what the post in post-AIDS can mean, as well as what the end in ending AIDS can mean. Firstly, post-AIDS discourses have often been invoked, it seems, as a way of talking about both a shift from fatal to chronic in terms of what it means to live with HIV. In this sense, post-AIDS takes on a specific medical connotation, that is, 'we are past the period when peopled died of AIDS'. Yet, we know that between 570,000 and 1.1 million people have died of AIDS-related illnesses as per UNAIDS 2018 report[1]. Post-AIDS narratives might also be invoked as a way of signaling the ushering in of ARV treatment, a discourse that is of course linked to the reduction of new AIDS cases. However, as Liz Walker has argued, to talk about a post-AIDS era belies the persistent stigmatization that is rampant across the globe for people living with HIV (Walker, 2017). I have touched upon this in my analysis of the concept of undetectability and the ethics of molecular HIV surveillance and, as such, the post in post-AIDS seems somewhat problematic. If post means 'that which comes after' something, and ending denotes the end of a period of time or a story, then post-AIDS and ending AIDS still seem to obscure the fact that there are chronic and persistent inequities across the globe, making the very notion of ending AIDS and a post-AIDS period problematic.

Perhaps then, the post in post-AIDS and the end in ending AIDS should signal something else. Informed by postcolonial studies, perhaps post-AIDS could entail a form of epistemology and even a praxeology. Rather than subscribing to the end of AIDS as a goal or as a time period, and moving away from post-AIDS as that which comes after 'AIDS crisis', we might think of the end of AIDS and post-AIDS as a set of discourses that describe ways of thinking and acting with, and in proximity to, HIV.

If epistemology is the study of how knowledge is generated, what methods are used and what theories are utilized in generating knowledge, then post-AIDS and ending AIDS has certainly been generative of several new ways of thinking through what it means to live with HIV, what risk means, what health means and what sexuality means (Guta, Murray, & Gagnon, 2016; Holt, 2014; Kenworthy et al., 2018; McClelland, Guta, & Gagnon, 2019; Persson, 2013, 2016; Persson, Newman, & Ellard, 2017; Persson, Newman, Mao, & de Wit, 2016).

Conversely, if praxeology is the study of human behavior and human action, then post-AIDS narratives and scholarship at the end of AIDS has certainly also generated a broad range of studies on how people act and engage in purposeful and meaningful actions not necessarily in the name of ending AIDS but as practices of sexuality, care, intimacy and wellbeing (Adam, 2006; Adam, Husbands, Murray, & Maxwell, 2005; Race, 2007, 2015, 2017). In this optic, the end of AIDS is not a process toward an ultimate goal, nor is it a time period; rather, it is a set of inquiries that are generated through the continual engagement with the very notion that we can, should and will end AIDS. Moving the lens from the end of AIDS as a time period or as an indicator-driven goal will perhaps allow us to see what the end of AIDS narrative obscures, what it forecloses, who is left behind and who is expected to end AIDS. Furthermore, it might allow us to move away from a strict biomedical discourse of what it means to end AIDS and rather engage with HIV as a generative and signifying epidemic that can tell us as much about power asymmetries, inequity and social issues as it can about biomedical metrics and technological inventions. Moreover, thinking about post-AIDS and ending AIDS as generative sets of epistemologies and praxeology allows us to also look at how people respond to, think through and act towards HIV not just as a problem of biomedicine, but also how meaning is generated, how intimacies are reconfigured and how notions of sexuality, pleasure and sociality are formed.

The notion that post-AIDS theory and theory generated in response to the signifying epidemic at the end of AIDS allows us, I think, to emphasize the importance of keeping track of and focusing on the dialectic relationship between both the continuities and the changes that have taken place within the HIV epidemic

(Kenworthy et al., 2018:967). Ending AIDS and the post-AIDS narrative as a set of epistemic and practical issues in response to HIV as a problem also allows us to see the epistemic continuities across the epidemic as Eileen Moyer has argued (Moyer, 2015). I have tried to show some of these continuities and differences. If Paula Treichler was looking for the dichotomies and signifying practices that merged in a period before ARVs, PrEP and molecular HIV mapping, I have tried to follow this with an optic that also seeks to tease out the novel and new, yet also the lingering and haunting within this signifying epidemic.

Ending AIDS seems to be a poly-vocal concept, which almost everyone can rally around, yet its ultimate meaning and how it will play out seem to be both contested and problematized. It has importantly meant an increasing reliance on biomedical technologies which, as Kane Race has warned us, might threaten to take the public out of public health (Race, 2009). This has been echoed by Susan Kippax and Niamh Stephenson as they worry that with increasing reliance on biomedical technologies, affected communities might lose their voice in the HIV effort (Kippax & Stephenson, 2016). This has been followed up by Vinh-Kim Nguyen as well (Nguyen, O'malley, & Pirkle, 2011). However, as I have shown in the case of emerging PrEP activism, new technologies also stir and rearrange activism, propels people to action and reconfigures what HIV activism is while also playing on older signifying practices which were present in the earlier days of the HIV epidemic.

While I share the skepticism of the aforementioned scholars toward a dogmatic and narrow biomedical end to AIDS, I think I have, in this book, also shown that resistance is also possible within this paradigm: resistance to focusing only on becoming undetectable, resistance to molecular HIV testing and resistance to being shamed for being on PrEP. The post in post-AIDS and the end in ending AIDS should perhaps be seen as processual and open rather than an event that seeks to put the final punctuation mark behind HIV and AIDS. Through resistance and the entanglements between new technologies and the social, new biosocialities are emerging, new norms are being negotiated and new forms of intimacies are being configured.

There is, of course, a danger in the encroachment of neoliberalism, austerity and a narrow biomedical focus, which we need to take seriously. As Leclerc-Madlala et al. state, it is important that the

> evidence base used in the HIV efforts are as inclusive and representative of the multiple dimensions of the human experience of HIV as possible. Against the near-total embrace of biomedical and big data approaches to ending AIDS, it is as if the narratives of people's lives are being swept away in the rapids of data streams and crushed under the weights of big data dashboards. This is not the imagery that a final triumph over AIDS should conjure.
> (Leclerc-Madlala, Broomhall, & Fieno, 2018:980)

My contribution to this has been to problematize the very notion of ending AIDS. I have tried to map some of how biomedical and biotechnological HIV sciences have come to produce new ways of signifying the end of AIDS. In this landscape, I have tried to attend to just the forms of imageries that are being conjured both in literal images and also in the images that are produced in HIV science on how to end AIDS. Seeing the end in ending AIDS and the post in post-AIDS as not solutions or goals, in and of themselves, I have rather tried to see them as productive problems in the signifying epidemic that is currently unfolding.

Attending to the future: speculation as method

I want to end with a few very brief statements on the future of the end of AIDS through a speculative method of inquiry. If my intended goal of this book was to problematize the end of AIDS and look into what this meant for HIV as an epidemic of signification, then these last pages will provide a speculative mapping of the possibilities of the future of the end of AIDS.

The first premise of this would be to acknowledge the limits of the current discourse of the end of AIDS. Take the UN SDGs and the notion that we will 'end the HIV epidemic' by 2030: projections and models abound in terms of how much funding is needed in this period, how many people need to be on ARVs and how many people need to be virally suppressed. Yet, these projections only allow for a temporal horizon that stretches to 2030. What then, of the time that lies beyond that horizon? Currently, between 32.7 million and 44 million people are living with HIV globally.[2] More and more people are living longer, healthier lives with HIV due to better access to ARVs as well as generally better health (Wing, 2016). In 2016, 10% of all people living with HIV were over 50 years old, and in the US, more than 50% of all people living with HIV were over 50 (Wing, 2016). Finally, it is projected that in 2030 70% of all people living with HIV in the US will be over 50 years of age (Wing, 2016). What does this mean for the notion of ending AIDS? Well from a biomedical standpoint we might argue that the goal is no more cases of AIDS. Yet, in light of these numbers, it seems to me that to talk about the end of AIDS as a temporally bound phenomenon with a set end date, and driven by a narrow biomedical treatment focus misses the mark of thinking holistically about living with HIV.

Ending AIDS, as it is currently being rolled out, has had some remarkable results. ARVs, PrEP and, to a certain degree, community-driven initiatives have been driving progress toward better, longer and healthier lives for more and more people. Yet, it also seems to be balancing on an edge between a biomedical doxa and human rights-driven initiatives. As increasing numbers of people are living longer, perhaps the end of AIDS needs to be seen as a more holistic ambition where the quality of life and human rights are given more space. Ending AIDS will entail the continued living with HIV, and, thankfully, more and more people will live long healthy lives. But this also means that we must lift our gaze beyond the 2030 horizon of the SDGs and acknowledge that we will have to cohabit and co-exist with HIV beyond the end of AIDS. The end of AIDS is not the end of HIV, and foreclosing the emergence of a vaccine or a cure, living with HIV will be part of our lives for the future. This is a fact that is not just a biomedical issue but also an issue within the socio-cultural realm of meaning-making. Affected communities have long lived with and in the proximity of HIV. It has been a history of dread, fear, suffering and death. However, it has also fueled activism, vitality, love, intimacies and political engagement like few other events in modern history. Cohabiting with this virus has been productive and will continue to be productive. Perhaps our task beyond the end of AIDS is to ensure that human rights are upheld, that communities and people living with and affected by HIV are involved in every step of the way toward the end of AIDS and beyond. The end of AIDS as a biomedical and bio-technological narrative needs to be supplemented by a narrative which focuses on the holistic lives of people living with HIV as well as the meaning-making generated in the entanglements between the biomedical, the technological and the social.

A second premise for the end of AIDS is, as Judith Auerbach has stated, to meaningfully engage with the 10-10-10 that currently are being left behind in the 90-90-90 targets (Auerbach, 2019). Judith Auerbach's important article has a thought-provoking title 'Getting to zero starts with getting to ten'. While I am not firmly against indicator-driven initiatives, I think Auerbach's title is illustrative of how the end of AIDS in the future should attend more to the gaps in the models and the lacuna in the indicators and acknowledge the need to grapple with the inequities that drive the HIV epidemic. The concern of the end of AIDS is that it will highlight only treatment pathways and not human rights pathways. The 10-10-10 is a good illustration of the embedded weakness of the end of AIDS if only seen as a mathematical problem to a social phenomenon. As such, the end of AIDS in the future needs to account for all people and their futures.

Much has changed during the course of the HIV epidemic since its start in 1981. Biomedical advances have led to people living long and healthy lives with HIV. Much has also changed in terms of the social context of the epidemic and the political economy that it is part of. Finally, there have been tremendous gains in human rights within certain spaces for people living with HIV. However, much work remains as still too many aspects of the end of AIDS remind us about the beginning of the AIDS epidemic. Stigma is still rampant globally, laws that punish same-sex practices are still an issue globally; so too are racism, homophobia and transphobia. Punitive HIV laws still exist and socioeconomic disparities are increasing.

With all of this, we need to think about the future of the HIV epidemic not as ending nor only as a biomedical problem to be solved. Rather we need to pay attention to the continuities between the beginning and the end of the HIV epidemic and how the end of AIDS is still also an epidemic of signification.

Notes

1 See UNAIDS fact sheet; https://www.unaids.org/en/resources/fact-sheet
2 See UNAIDS fact sheet; https://www.unaids.org/en/resources/fact-sheet

References

Adam, B. D. (2006). Infectious behavior: Imputing subjectivity to HIV transmission. *Social Theory and Health*, *4*(2), 168–179.

Adam, B. D., Husbands, W., Murray, J., & Maxwell, J. (2005). AIDS optimism, condom fatigue, or self-esteem? Explaining unsafe sex among gay and bisexual men. *Journal of Sex Research*, *42*(3), 238–248.

Auerbach, J. D. (2019). Getting to zero begins with getting to ten. *Journal of Acquired Immune Deficiency Syndromes (1999)*, *82*(2), S99.

Baum, C., Birenbaum-Carmeli, D., Ferzacca, S., Frank, G., Good, B., Hall-Clifford, R. … Wiedman, D. (2010). Chronic conditions, fluid states: Chronicity and the anthropology of illness. Retrieved from https://www.degruyter.com/isbn/9780813549736.

Bhabha, H. K. (2012). *The location of culture*. London: Routledge.

Dimitris, S., Edwards, O., Hull, B., Margolese, S., Mason, N., Namiba, A. … Ross, G. V. (2012). Language, identity, and HIV: Why do we keep talking about the responsible and responsive use of language? Language matters. *Journal of the International AIDS Society*, *15*, 17990.

Fanon, F. (2008). *Black skin, white masks*. New York, NY: Grove press.

Guta, A., Murray, S. J., & Gagnon, M. (2016). HIV, viral suppression and new technologies of surveillance and control. *Body & Society*, *22*(2), 82–107.

Holt, M. (2014). Gay men's HIV risk reduction practices: The influence of epistemic communities in HIV social and behavioral research. *AIDS Education and Prevention*, *26*(3), 214–223.

Kenworthy, N., Thomann, M., & Parker, R. (2018). From a global crisis to the 'end of AIDS': New epidemics of signification. *Global Public Health*, *13*(8), 960–971.

Kippax, S., & Stephenson, N. (2016). *Socializing the biomedical turn in HIV prevention*. New York, NY: Anthem Press.

Leclerc-Madlala, S., Broomhall, L., & Fieno, J. (2018). The 'end of AIDS'project: Mobilising evidence, bureaucracy, and big data for a final biomedical triumph over AIDS. *Global Public Health*, *13*(8), 972–981.

Ledin, C. W., & Benjamin (2019). PrEP at the after/Party: The 'post-AIDS' politics of Frank ocean's "PrEP+". *Somatosphere*. Published online.

Lewis, N. M., Bauer, G. R., Coleman, T. A., Blot, S., Pugh, D., Fraser, M., & Powell, L. (2015). Community cleavages: Gay and bisexual men's perceptions of gay and mainstream community acceptance in the post-AIDS, post-rights era. *Journal of Homosexuality*, *62*(9), 1201–1227.

Loomba, A. (2007). *Colonialism/postcolonialism*. London: Routledge.

McClelland, A., Guta, A., & Gagnon, M. (2019). The rise of molecular HIV surveillance: Implications on consent and criminalization. *Critical Public Health*, 1–7.

Moyer, E. (2015). The anthropology of life after AIDS: Epistemological continuities in the age of antiretroviral treatment. *Annual Review of Anthropology*, *44*(1), 259–275.

Nguyen, V.-K., O'malley, J., & Pirkle, C. M. (2011). Remedicalizing an epidemic: From HIV treatment as prevention to HIV treatment is prevention. *AIDS*, *25*(11), 1435.

Persson, A. (2013). Non/infectious corporealities: Tensions in the biomedical era of 'HIV normalization'. *Sociology of Health and Illness*, *35*(7), 1065–1079.

Persson, A. (2016). 'The world has changed': Pharmaceutical citizenship and the reimagining of serodiscordant sexuality among couples with mixed HIV status in Australia. *Sociology of Health and Illness*, *38*(3), 380–395.

Persson, A., Newman, C. E., & Ellard, J. (2017). Breaking binaries? Biomedicine and serostatus borderlands among couples with mixed HIV status. *Medical Anthropology, 36*(8), 699–713.

Persson, A., Newman, C. E., Mao, L., & de Wit, J. (2016). On the margins of pharmaceutical citizenship: Not taking HIV medication in the "treatment revolution" era. *Medical Anthropology Quarterly, 30*(3), 359–377.

Race, K. (2007). Engaging in a culture of barebacking: Gay men and the risk of HIV prevention. In Mark Davis and Corinne Squire (Eds.), *HIV Treatment and Prevention Technologies in International Perspective* (pp. 107–134). London: Palgrave Macmillan.

Race, K. (2009). *Pleasure consuming medicine: The queer politics of drugs*. Durham: Duke University Press.

Race, K. (2015). 'Party and play': Online hook-up devices and the emergence of PNP practices among gay men. *Sexualities, 18*(3), 253–275.

Race, K. (2017). *The gay science: Intimate experiments with the problem of HIV*. London: Routledge.

Rofes, E. (2015). *Dry bones breathe: Gay men creating post-AIDS identities and cultures*. London: Routledge.

Said, E. W. (2003). *Orientalism* (Repr., with a new preface. ed.). London: Penguin Books.

Sangaramoorthy, T. (2018). Chronicity, crisis, and the 'end of AIDS'. *Global Public Health, 13*(8), 982–996.

Spivak, G. C. (1999). *A critique of postcolonial reason: Toward a history of the vanishing present*. Cambridge, MA: Harvard university press.

Treichler, P. A. (1999). *How to have theory in an epidemic: Cultural Chronicles of AIDS*. Durham: Duke University Press.

Tung, Warren, & Jungwirth, Barbara (2017). This week in HIV research Stable housing improves viral suppression and CD4 counts. *The BodyPro*. Retrieved from https://www.thebodypro.com/article/this-week-in-hiv-research-stable-housing-improves-.

UNAIDS. (2010). *Getting to zero: 2011–2015 Strategy*. Geneva: World Health Organization.

Vigh, H. (2008). Crisis and chronicity: Anthropological perspectives on continuous conflict and decline. *Ethnos, 73*(1), 5–24.

Walker, L. (2017). Problematizing the discourse of 'post-AIDS'. *Journal of Medical Humanities*, 1–11.

Wing, E. J. (2016). HIV and aging. *International Journal of Infectious Diseases, 53*, 61–68.

Index

Printed in the United States
by Baker & Taylor Publisher Services